THE SHAMBHALA GUIDE TO
TRADITIONAL CHINESE MEDICINE

The
Shambhala Guide to
TRADITIONAL
CHINESE
MEDICINE

Daniel Reid

SHAMBHALA
Boston & London
1996

Shambhala Publications, Inc.
Horticultural Hall
300 Massachusetts Avenue
Boston, Massachusetts 02115

9 8 7 6 5 4 3 2 1

First Edition
Printed in the United States of America
⊗ This edition is printed on acid-free paper that meets
the American National Standards Institute Z39.48 Standard.
Distributed in the United States by Random House, Inc.,
and in Canada by Random House of Canada Ltd

Library of Congress Cataloging-in-Publication Data

Reid, Daniel P., 1948–
    The Shambhala guide to traditional Chinese medicine
  /by Daniel Reid.
       p.   cm.
    ISBN 1-57062-141-1 (alk. paper)
    1. Medicine, Chinese.   I. Title.
  R602.R45   1996   95-23897
  610'.951—dc20   CIP

For my aunt Ilse and my brother Fred

Contents

THE SHAMBHALA GUIDE TO
TRADITIONAL CHINESE MEDICINE

Introduction

IN TRADITIONAL CHINESE MEDICINE, the human system is viewed as a microcosmic mirror of the macrocosmic universe, a whole inner world composed of the same elements and energies, and subject to the same natural laws, as the external world and cosmos (fig. 1). The universal principles that govern "everything under Heaven" (*tien hsia*) are simply known as the "Way" (Tao), and they apply equally to stars and planets, molecules and atoms, operating exactly the same way in the human system as they do in the solar system. Because nature is the most obvious and enduring manifestation of Tao on earth, much of the traditional terminology of Chinese medicine is derived directly from natural phenomena (fire and water, wind and heat, dryness and dampness, etc.), and a traditional Chinese diagnosis often sounds more like a weather report than a medical analysis. In Chinese medicine, manifest nature is the master template by which the physician understands and manipulates the internal elements and energies of the human system.

When the elemental energies within the human system remain in a natural state of dynamic balance and functional harmony, "fair weather" prevails inside the body, and the garden of human health flourishes, both mentally and physically. But when organic balance

1

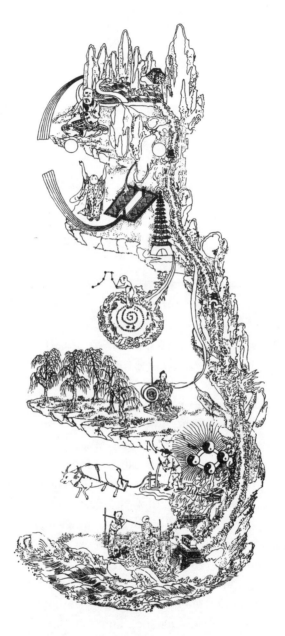

Figure 1. An ancient Chinese depiction of the human system as a microcosm of nature and the cosmos.

is upset and aberrant energies invade the system, flood and drought, wind and rain, heat and cold, and other types of "stormy weather" may occur, causing damage to the internal landscape. Because the microcosmic energy system of humans (*ren*) stands midway between the cosmic powers of Heaven (*tien*) and the natural forces of Earth (*di*), drawing power from both sources, human health depends not only on internal energy balance within the system, but also on harmony with the macrocosmic powers of Heaven (the cosmos) and Earth (nature).

Two key concepts in traditional Chinese medicine are that the occurrence of disease represents a failure in preventive health care, and that health is a responsibility shared equally by doctor and patient. In the Chinese medical tradition, the doctor serves mainly as advisor and guide, the coach who teaches the patient the basic ground rules and winning strategies in the game of health, but it is up to each individual to play the game and win or lose the prize of health. The key tactic in the game of health is timing and preventive intervention. As the classic verse of the *Tao Teh Ching* states,

> Before an omen arises,
> It's easy to take preventive measures . . .
> Deal with things in their formative state;
> Put things in order before they grow confused.

The traditional Chinese approach to health is summarized in the old English adage, "A stitch in time saves nine." The Chinese have always realized the wisdom of spending time and money on a preventive stitch now, rather than having to pay the pain and cost of nine curative stitches later. That is one reason that Chinese in all walks of life rarely stint on expenditures for food: they learned long ago that you are what you eat, and they know that wholesome food is always the best preventive medicine. In the Western world today, people tend to take health for granted until it breaks down, then run to the doctor looking for a quick fix or a spare part. "Such an approach," states *The Yellow Emperor's Classic of Internal Medicine*, "is comparable to the behavior of a person who starts digging a well only after he is thirsty, or who begins to forge weapons after he is already engaged in battle. Would these actions not be too late?"

"The superior physician," says an old Chinese medical axiom, "teaches his patients how to stay healthy." In traditional Chinese households, the family doctor was retained not just to treat the sick but to keep everyone in the family, including the servants, healthy. The physician visited the household regularly, checking everyone's pulse and other vital signs and dispensing timely advice and remedies as required in order to deal with things in their formative state. As long as everyone in the household remained healthy, the doctor received a regular monthly fee, but if anyone fell ill, all payments stopped until the doctor restored the patient to health, at the doctor's own expense! Not only was this system an excellent preventive against disease, it was also a very effective preventive against malpractice and a strong incentive to creative progress in health care, for the income of physicians depended entirely on keeping their clients healthy, not on treating them for diseases that could easily have been prevented with "a stitch in time," as is all too often the case in modern Western medicine.

Traditional Chinese doctors diagnose and treat the whole human system, rather than dealing only with its separate parts, as the specialists of modern Western medicine do. Western medicine tends to focus on the overt symptoms of disease in the part of the body where they occur, treating each condition in the same way in every patient, as though the symptom were an independent phenomenon unrelated to other parts of the body and the external environment. The Chinese describe this sort of medical care as suppressing the superficial symptoms while failing to cure the root cause. By contrast, Chinese medicine diagnoses and treats all symptoms of disease in terms of their functional relationships to the whole human system, as well as to external factors in the environment in which the symptoms developed. Primary attention is always focused on the subtle governing energies that operate decisively below the surface, not on the obvious external symptoms they create outside. This is called "curing the root, not treating the surface."

The Chinese view the human body as an organic system whose parts are all functionally interrelated by virtue of the same fundamental forces that govern nature and the cosmos, of which the human system is a microcosmic but complete reflection. As Ted Kaptchuk explains in *The Web That Has No Weaver*,

> To Western medicine, understanding an illness means uncovering a distinct entity that is separate from the patient's being; to Chinese medicine, understanding means perceiving the relationships between all the patient's signs and symptoms. . . . The Chinese method is thus holistic, based on the idea that no single part can be understood except in its relation to the whole. . . . If a person has a symptom, Chinese medicine wants to know how the symptom fits into the patient's entire bodily pattern. . . . Understanding that overall pattern, with the symptom as part of it, is the challenge of Chinese medicine.

In Western medicine, the human body is seen as a machine consisting of many separate, often replaceable parts, and the doctor is a specialized mechanic who fixes the machine when it stalls, or replaces worn-out parts when it breaks down. Prior to the actual onset of disease, modern Western medicine doesn't tend to emphasize regular preventive health care. And some modern Western therapies, such as surgery, radiation, chemotherapy, and chemical drugs, are highly intrusive and sometimes toxic to the human system, often doing damage to the body that only manifests years later, when it is diagnosed and treated as an entirely different disease. Chinese medicine views the human body as a flourishing living garden and the doctor as a gardener who periodically trims, prunes, weeds, waters, fertilizes, and takes care of the various organisms to prevent the whole garden from withering and going to seed. The doctor uses wholesome foods, herbs, acupuncture, massage, exercise, and other natural, nonintrusive methods to cultivate the whole human garden and protect it from damage by the aberrant forces of nature. While modern Western medicine employs technology as a weapon of war against the forces of nature involved in human disease, with the body as a battlefield, Chinese medicine tries to harness, harmonize, and deflect malevolent energies to rebalance and retune the whole human system. The Chinese way slowly but surely restores the human system to a state of equilibrium, thereby eliminating the symptoms that inevitably arise whenever human energies lose their internal balance and fall out of harmony with the environmental forces of Heaven and Earth.

One of the problems with modern Western medicine is that it developed largely on the basis of dissection and study of cadavers, and this research has been literally applied to living human beings, without taking adequate account for the dynamic energies that govern the physical organs and other parts of living human bodies. This has led to a strong mechanical and chemical bias in modern Western medical practice, and insufficient attention to the vital roles played by the invisible but decisive forces of energy within the human system. In Chinese medicine, however, the human energy system has always been regarded as the key factor in health and healing.

The eighteenth-century Japanese medical commentator Mitani Kolu tellingly observed: "As Western medicine studies more and more detail, it moves further away from the real aim of its research. . . . Its studies of the human body concern only the cadaver. They do not inform us about the living, the only true aim of medical studies."

The Chinese view human beings in terms of three inseparable, interpenetrating dimensions of existence, called the Three Treasures (*san bao*): these are *jing* (essence, body), *chee* (energy, breath), and *shen* (spirit, mind). These distinctly different but totally interdependent aspects of human life are equivalent to the Tibetan Buddhist concept of the three *kaya*: *dharmakaya* (dimension of mind), *sambhogakaya* (dimension of energy), and *nirmanakaya* (dimension of body). The Three Treasures compose the framework of human existence, the foundation of human life, and the basic ingredients in the "internal alchemy" (*nei-gung*) of traditional Taoist meditation, medicine, and martial arts. An ancient Taoist text entitled *Classification of Therapies* states, "Essence transforms into energy, and energy transforms into spirit." This process of transformation and sublimation of energy is the basis of Taoist internal alchemy and is achieved by applying the corollary to the above equation, "Spirit commands energy, and energy commands essence." Known as the Triplex Unity, this formula means that the mind controls energy and energy controls the body to ensure that the body produces energy and energy sustains the mind (fig. 2).

Jing refers to the physical body, particularly its "vital essence,"

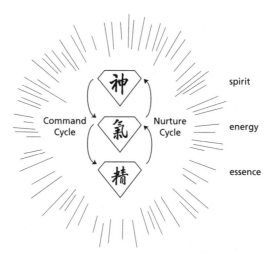

Figure 2. Taoist internal alchemy of the Triplex Unity of Essence, Energy, and Spirit, with the nurture and command cycles for internal balance and harmony.

such as blood, hormones, enzymes, lymph, immune factors, and other essential bodily components. *Chee* refers to the sum total of all the vital energies within the human system, and also to the constituent energies of each internal organ, gland, tissue, and other functional part. *Shen* refers to pure primordial spirit as well as to the temporal aspects of spirit that define the human mind in all its various facets and functions. The Three Treasures of life are only one aspect of a basic dimensional trinity—along with the Three Powers (Heaven, Earth, Humanity) and the Three Elixir Fields (navel, solar plexus, head)—that runs throughout traditional Chinese philosophy, fusing the three major Taoist practices of meditation, medicine, and martial arts into one unified system. Internal balance on each level of existence—physical, energetic, and mental—and harmony among all three are the keys to human health and longevity.

Western medicine recognizes only soma (the body, or *jing*) and psyche (the mind, or *shen*), dividing them into two separate and often antagonistic departments of health care (physiology and psychology), then further fragmenting various aspects of each into even more specialized subdepartments, with little or no cross-referencing. In the Western view, the physical body reigns supreme, with energy seen as a mere byproduct of physiological metabolism and consciousness as an outgrowth of the brain. To the Chinese, however, the spirit and its various facets of awareness and volition are the primary governing factors in human life, whereas energy is regarded as the basic self-existing fuel of the universe, which spirit harnesses to accomplish its purposes, and the body is simply condensed energy organized by the human mind to form a physical vehicle for manifest life on earth. Not only are these two views of human life fundamentally different in philosophy, they also give rise to very different approaches to human health and disease in medical practice.

According to the Chinese view, the mind may be engaged to control and guide energy to heal and repair the body. Western medical science has recently confirmed this view with the discovery of the so-called psychoneuroimmunology (PNI) response, through which positive states of mind such as compassion, love, faith, calm, happiness, and so forth generate specific healing responses in the body. They are thought to do this by stimulating secretions of the particular hormones and neurochemicals involved in immunity and healing. Conversely, negative thoughts and emotions like anger, grief, jealousy, hatred, and stress generate essences and energies that inhibit immune response, unbalance the system, and fling open the gates to disease and degeneration.

Conventional Western medicine separates ailments of body and mind, turning physical problems over to physicians and surgeons and mental and emotional problems to psychologists and psychiatrists. Neither one deals with nor even understands the underlying human energies that link physical and mental symptoms in a unified, organically integrated system, and therefore neither can provide a cure that heals both body and mind and restores a healthy equilibrium to the whole human system. Chinese medicine deals directly with the underlying imbalances and dysfunctions of energy that lie at the root of both physiological and psychological symptoms of disease, thereby curing the whole system with the same therapies. An interesting and beneficial side effect of traditional Chinese therapy is that, in balancing and healing the mind as well as the body, it often leaves the patient at the doorstep of spiritual discovery, and many patients go on to take up meditation, *chee-gung* (also spelled *qigong* or *ch'i-kung*) and other traditional Chinese methods of total self-health cultivation.

Both in theory and in practice, *chee*, and its various roles in the human system, lies at the very heart of traditional Chinese medicine. Invisible and immaterial, *chee* is nevertheless the most basic component of life, the formative force behind all manifest existence, and the motive power that drives all activities and catalyzes all transformations, mental and emotional as well as physical. The essential nature of this vital energy remains one of life's great mysteries, yet its effects are apparent and tangible, and its powers and properties are easily perceived and understood by what it does in nature and within the human system. Miraculous in its infinite potency and pervasive presence throughout all realms of nature and the universe, *chee* manifests its decisive power over matter in everything from the formation and dissolution of stars and galaxies down to the most mundane phenomena of nature on earth—a falling leaf, a rotting apple, a self-replicating cell, a waterfall, a burp, or a sneeze. It is the beat in the heart, the warmth in the blood, the rhythmic expansion and contraction of breath. *Chee* is both the cause and the effect of every activity and phenomenon in atoms, molecules, cells, organs, bodies, planets, stars, galaxies, and the universe as a whole.

In *The Web That Has No Weaver*, Ted Kaptchuk writes, "The tendency of Chinese thought is to seek out dynamic functional activity rather than to look for fixed somatic structures that perform activities." The primacy of energy over matter, function over form, is one of the most distinctive hallmarks of traditional Chinese medicine. For all the detailed precision of Western anatomical and physiological science, modern Western medicine still lacks a comprehensive and systematic view of the vital forces that forge matter, shape form, and drive all functions in the human body, weaving the invisible web of energy that constitutes the master blueprint for all physical structures in the body and controls the activities of the whole system and all its parts. The patterns of the human energy system are woven by both Heaven (cosmic energies) and Earth (natural forces), and they are permanently encoded in the filaments of DNA within each and every cell of the body. Distortions in human energy patterns are always the primary cause of disease and degeneration, and such distortions are in turn caused by exposure to aberrant external or unbalanced internal energies.

Chinese medicine views physical disease as being the final symptomatic manifestation of long-standing imbalances, deficiencies, obstructions, and other chronic abnormalities in the flow and patterns of the human energy system, and it cures disease by restoring and rebalancing disordered internal energies and reestablishing energetic harmony with the environment. As soon as normal balance and harmony are restored to the energy system, it immediately goes to work repairing physical damage, eliminating toxins, replacing cells, and rebuilding tissues—all according to the master plan contained in DNA, the body's most effective prescription for health and longevity. One of the keys to Chinese preventive medicine is to detect and correct abnormal patterns in the human energy system before they become somatically rooted in the body and cause permanent physical damage.

A major reason for the megacrisis in human health throughout the world today is the fact that modern urban lifestyles and industrial technology have isolated and alienated humanity from the powers of nature and the cosmos, the context in which human life has evolved in harmony for millions of years. A basic tenet of the holistic organic view of humanity, nature, and the cosmos is that whatever benefits the whole also benefits all its constituent parts. Although modern American medicine does not share the holistic view of Chinese medicine, traditional Native American views on human health show remarkable similarities to the Chinese approach, as evidenced in this memorable statement by Chief Seattle in 1854:

> The earth does not belong to man; man belongs to the earth.
> All things are connected. . . . What befalls the earth befalls
> the sons of the earth. Man did not weave the web of life; he
> is merely a strand in it. Whatever he does to the web, he
> does to himself.

When humanity pollutes the air with toxic smog and fills the sky with microwaves, artificial electromagnetic fields, and other abnormal energies, and when we poison the soil and waters with toxic chemicals and foul wastes, we also distort the energies, poison the fluids, and pollute the tissues of our own internal worlds. Humanity simply cannot have it both ways: we cannot derange and denature the macrocosm of our living environment without deranging and destroying the microcosm of life within ourselves.

By promoting and protecting the primordial purity, natural balance, and inherent harmony of the Three Powers of Heaven, Earth, and Humanity, and integrating them with the Three Treasures of body, energy, and mind, we can just as easily prevent disease, arrest degeneration, and prolong life as we can destroy health and hasten death through ignorance and violation of the natural laws that govern life on earth. All that life really requires to accomplish the goals of health and longevity is to synchronize its energies with the natural pulses of the planet and the rhythms of the cosmos from which life springs. Traditional Chinese medicine endeavors to facilitate this harmonic balance on all three levels of body, energy, and mind with nutrition, herbs, acupuncture, massage, *chee-gung*, meditation, and other holistic methods that restore nature's patterns to the human energy system and weave it back into its proper position in the great web of life on earth.

1
Historical Milestones in Chinese Medicine

TRADITIONAL CHINESE MEDICINE is rooted in the very foundations of Chinese civilization, the cornerstones of which were laid in the Central Plain of the Yellow River Basin in northern China at least five thousand years ago. While Western scholars still tend to discount this formative period of Chinese history as "mythical," and refer to the founding emperor Huang Ti (the Yellow Emperor) as "legendary," recent archeological excavations in China have finally confirmed the existence of a major civilization that flourished in the Yellow River basin around 3000 BCE, governed by an emperor named Huang Ti. Virtually every historical record and archeological discovery in China dating from this early formative period down to the present time has testified to the central importance of medicine in Chinese civilization.

Prior to the advent of professional physicians during the early Chou dynasty (1122–249 BCE), Chinese medicine was the exclusive domain of tribal shamans (*wu*). These "medicine men" collected the wild herbs brought down from the mountains of ancient China by wandering Taoist hermits, tested and categorized them, and used them for healing. This was the era of the emperor Shen Nung (the "Divine Farmer"), who, according to the authoritative Han dynasty historian Ssu Ma-chien, "tasted the myriad herbs, and so the art of medicine was born." References to thirty-six different diseases and their herbal cures have been found inscribed on some of the 160,000 tortoise shells and oracle bones excavated during the twentieth century in the Central Plain region, dating mainly from the ancient Yin dynasty, circa 1500 BCE. This proves that disease and medicine had already become a systematic field of study in China, if not an actual profession, as long as thirty-five hundred years ago.

During the Chou dynasty, which replaced the Yin in 1122 BCE, Chinese language and civilization underwent rapid development, and the art of medicine began to detach itself from its former association with sorcery and superstition. The ancient Chinese ideogram for "doctor" (*yi*) first appeared in written records dating from the early Chou era, indicating that medicine had already become an independent profession, no longer a branch of shamanism. The ideogram for "medicine" (*yao*) also made its first appearance in classical records of the early Chou period.

The terms *yi* and *yao* appear frequently in the *I-Ching* (*Book of Change*), the world's oldest extant book. This ancient Chinese canon of philosophy and divination was written during the twelfth century BCE by the duke of Chou and represents the earliest recorded codification of the ancient edifice of Taoist philosophy on which all the traditional Chinese arts and sciences are founded. The terms *yin* and *yang* also made their first appearance in written form in the beguiling text of the *I-Ching*, as in the following passage:

> The ceaseless interplay of Heaven [cosmos] and Earth [nature] gives forms to all things. The sexual union of male and female gives life to all things. This interaction of yin and yang is called Tao [the Way], and the resulting creative process is called change.

In 218 BCE, the militant kingdom of Chin, from which the West derived the name *China*, swept down from the northwest and conquered all the warring kingdoms and squabbling principalities that had arisen to fill the vacuum left by the decline and fall of the ancient Chou dynasty, uniting the entire empire under a single centralized government for the first time in Chinese history. In his ruthless drive to eradicate all vestiges of the past, the first Chin emperor ordered the infamous Fires of Chin, a mass book-burning campaign in which virtually all written records of ancient China's classical heritage went up in flames. The only exceptions to this wholesale destruction of recorded knowledge were books on agriculture, divination (including the *I-Ching*), and medicine.

After enduring the cruelty of Chin rule for fifteen years, the Chinese people revolted and passed the Mandate of Heaven to the great Han dynasty (206 BCE–220 CE), under which Chinese civilization as we know it today took on its distinctive form and character. The early Han and the preceding Warring States periods were times of great intellectual ferment in China, and many of the most important Chinese philosophers, from Confucius and Mencius to Lao Tze and Chuang Tze, appeared during these centuries, along with the classical texts written by or attributed to them. Early Han authors wrote three important medical texts that for the first time organized the vast body of medical experience accumulated in China during the previous three millennia, and these became the first classic canons of traditional Chinese medicine.

The most important of these early Han medical texts was entitled *The Yellow Emperor's Classic of Internal Medicine* (*Huang Ti Nei Ching*), and today it remains an indispensable text in the study of traditional Chinese medicine. Like many other Han classics, this title carries the name of one of China's most venerated ancient emperors to enhance its aura of authority, as though the text had flowed directly from the brush of that august source, but in fact it was compiled during the early Han. This book sifted science from superstition and elucidated the essential guiding principles of traditional Chinese medicine, establishing a systematic theoretical framework for the study and practice of medicine as a profession. The text explains the practical medical applications of the Great Principle of Yin and Yang, the Five Elemental Energies, and other primordial principles of Taoist philosophy, and many of the therapeutics it introduced are still applied in clinical practice today. (There are two English translations of this medical canon, listed in the bibliography.)

Another famous Han medical classic is *The Pharmacopeia of Shen Nung (Shen Nung Pen Tsao Ching)*, which recorded all the knowledge on medicinal herbs handed down in China from previous eras, separating fact from fancy and including only clinically proven claims. Shen Nung was the ancient Chinese emperor to whom the Han historian Ssu Ma-chien attributed the birth of Chinese medicine. The Han pharmacopeia that carries his name divides all known medicinal herbs into three functional categories: the "upper" class nurtures life and promotes longevity; the "middle" group nurtures nature and bestows vitality; the "lower" category was labeled "poison" and included all toxic herbs used to combat the most virulent infectious diseases. These categories still stand in Chinese herbal medicine today.

The third great medical treatise of the early Han was called *Discussion of Fevers and Flus (Shang Han Lun)*, written by Chang Chung-ching around 200 BCE. Over half of Dr. Chang's own clan had died of various types of fevers, prompting him to devote his life to the study of cures for these ailments. He divided all diseases into six types—three yin and three yang—and his prescriptions were formulated to correct imbalances in the polar yin/yang forces of the human system, thereby curing the root causes of disease in the body. Dr. Chang also wrote another milestone medical treatise entitled *Essential Prescriptions of the Golden Chest*. Originally this and *Shang Han Lun* were combined into one book, but later they were divided into two separate volumes. In addition, he produced and published the first map of the energy meridians and vital points used in acupuncture. His book, which today is still respected as an authoritative classic reference manual for preparing herbal formulas, lists 113 medical prescriptions employing 100 herbs. Some of his formulas have long been used as tried-and-true folk remedies handed down from generation to generation in Chinese families, such as Cinnamon Sap Soup, which contains cinnamon, ginger, licorice, jujubes, and peony, and is still used as a remedy for fevers with chills in Chinese medicine. (An English translation of and commentary on *Shang Han Lun* is listed in the bibliography.)

During the late Han (25–220 CE), there appeared another great physician who left his permanent personal imprint on traditional Chinese medicine. His name was Hua To (140–208 CE), and he was the first to use toxic herbs such as *Datura metel, Rhododendron sinense,* and *Aconitum* to induce local anesthesia prior to topical surgery. There is a famous painting depicting Hua To performing surgery to remove a poisoned arrowhead embedded in the arm of the great historical hero General Kuan Yu, who was later deified as the Chinese god of war. Thanks to the doctor's herbal painkiller, the stoic general was able calmly to play chess with a fellow officer while Hua To scraped away the infected flesh in his arm, right down to the bone. Hua To is also well remembered for the set of therapeutic exercises called *dao-yin,* which he developed and prescribed for various illnesses, based on the movements of animals. *Dao-yin,* which means "to induce and guide" (as to induce and guide energy through the body), is still taught and practiced as health therapy in China today.

In 629 CE, the founding emperor of the great Tang dynasty (618–906 CE), known as China's Golden Age, issued a decree commanding that all medical knowledge in the empire should henceforth be collected and codified in the capital of Chang An (present-day Sian), where he established China's first school of medicine. The Tang produced a number of famous physicians, some of whom recorded their knowledge in texts that have since joined the ranks of Chinese medical classics. The Tang herbalist Tao Hung-ching wrote two books entitled *Herbs as Studied by Shen Nung* (*Shen Nung Tsao Yao Hsueh*) and *Anecdotes of Celebrated Physicians* (*Ming Yi Ku Shih*), in which he compiled and commented on medical data handed down from previous eras.

By far the most renowned physician of the Tang era, and one of the most important figures in the history of Chinese medicine, was Sun Ssu-miao (590–692 CE). Dr. Sun turned down requests by two Tang emperors to become their personal physician so that he could continue his private practice and medical research among the common people. He lived to the age of 101 by practicing what he preached, and he preached what he practiced by writing the great medical compendium entitled *Precious Recipes* (*Chian Chin Fang*), which contains valuable information and commentary on every aspect of traditional Chinese health care, including herbs and acupuncture, diet and exercise, breathing, and sexual yoga. This book contains the earliest Chinese references to diseases of nutritional deficiency, such as beri beri and scurvy, which he correctly diagnosed and successfully treated with nutrient remedies. He identified goiter, for example, as being caused by lack of a vital nutrient (iodine) in the diets of those who live far from the sea, and he cured the condition by prescribing seaweed and extracts of deer and lamb thyroid, all of which are rich dietary sources of iodine. *Precious Recipes* constitutes one of the most comprehensive practical handbooks of traditional Chinese medicine and includes chapters on Taoist sexual yoga and longevity practices as well.

During the ensuing Sung dynasty (960–1279 CE), Chinese medicine continued to advance rapidly, and several new medical schools were established in China. Medical students were now required to treat ailing faculty members, government officials, and military officers as part of their training, and the results were included in their final examination scores for graduation. All herbal prescriptions throughout the empire were standardized, and new forms of herbal medicine, such as poultices, pills, and patent formulas, appeared in practice. The official imperial pharmacopeia of medical herbs was revised and expanded four times, the last edition listing almost one thousand items.

After a brief period of dormancy during the Mongol Yuan dynasty (1260–1368 CE), Chinese medicine once again took a great leap forward under the native Ming (1368–1644), during which classical Chinese culture enjoyed a flourishing renaissance. The Ming produced another great master of Chinese herbal medicine, Li Shih-chen (1517–1593), who spent twenty-seven years of his life compiling and writing the book that has become the single most authoritative pharmacopeia of Chinese herbal medicine, *Outlines and Divisions of Herbal Medicine (Pen Tsao Kang Mu)*. Contained in fifty-two book-scrolls listing 1,892 medicinal plants, minerals, and animal products, this great materia medica has become the bible of Chinese herbalists throughout the world and remains an indispensable reference in the study and practice of Chinese medicine. It has also been translated in its entirety into Japanese, Korean, Vietnamese, French, German, Russian, and English, and was the first Chinese medical text to be seriously accepted and studied in the West, where it is said to have had an important influence on Charles Darwin's theories of evolution. An English translation, by G. A. Stuart and B. E. Read, was published in three volumes in Shanghai in 1911 and has been reprinted in Taiwan (see bibliography).

Li Shih-chen was the last great giant in the classical history of Chinese medicine. During the following Manchu Ching dynasty (1644–1911), the study and practice of the Chinese healing arts continued unabated and enjoyed particularly generous imperial patronage, and many important texts on specific branches of Chinese medicine were written and published, but very few have been fully translated into English. This period, which first brought China and the West into close contact, also saw many Chinese medicinal herbs find their way into British, American, and European pharmacopeias, where they sowed the first seeds of the hybrid "New Medicine" that is now fusing traditional Eastern and modern Western medical practices in many parts of the world today.

While many traditional medical systems have long since fallen into disuse because of competition from modern Western medical technology, traditional Chinese medicine still dominates the field of health in China, where it now continues to evolve and expand in conjunction rather than competition with modern medical science. The inevitable showdown between Chinese and Western medicine took place in Shanghai back in 1929, but unlike so many other conflicts between past and present ways, the traditionalists won the day in Chinese medicine, much to the everlasting benefit of China's national health.

At that time, young Chinese doctors newly trained in Japan in the wonders of modern Western medicine had just returned to China and were loudly clamoring for traditional medicine to be legally banned as an archaic and superstitious remnant of the past. This provoked such adamant opposition from all quarters of Chinese society that an extraordinary meeting of the most renowned traditional physicians in China was convened in Shanghai, and they elected a delegation to plead their case to the Nationalist government in nearby Nanking. After due consideration (no doubt many elder Nationalist leaders had personally experienced the benefits of Chinese medicine), the government declared its full support for traditional Chinese medicine on March 17, and ever since that milestone decision, which saved Chinese medicine from extinction in the dustbin of history, this date has been celebrated in China as Chinese Doctor Day. Two years later, in 1931, the League of Nations established a special committee in Geneva to undertake a comprehensive study of traditional Chinese medicine, thereby bringing the ancient healing arts of China under modern scientific investigation in the laboratories of the Western world.

Since then, Western medical science has confirmed many of the theories and validated many of the practices of traditional Chinese medicine, and numerous Western scholars and scientists have devoted their entire professional careers to the study and practice of this ancient health system. (A selection of the more important books written by Western scholars and practitioners of Chinese medicine are included in the bibliography.)

Meanwhile, in the medical clinics and scientific laboratories of China, Hong Kong, Taiwan, Japan, and Korea, as well as in Western countries where Chinese medicine has been accepted, traditional Chinese therapeutics are being submitted to rigorous scientific testing, and exciting new discoveries are being made every year, including safe and effective herbal birth control, cures for AIDS and cancer, electronically enhanced acupuncture, new herbal cures for drug-resistant strains of malaria and other deadly diseases, and much more. These discoveries are all being incorporated in the New Medicine, which blends the best of East and West in human health and healing and offers new hope for resolution of medical mysteries that neither traditional nor modern medicine alone has been able to solve.

When it comes to medicine, what really counts is how well it works in practice, not how well it accords with this or that theory, and this is something only patients can testify to with certainty. It was the spontaneous testimony of millions of patients in China that saved traditional medicine from being abolished by its modern detractors in 1929, and it remains the trust and confidence of hundreds of millions of patients throughout the world that allows this ancient way of health to continue developing today.

2
The Human Energy System

The human energy system is like an electric power plant that runs in patterned circuits through each and every functional part of a complex machine or factory, delivering and regulating the current which controls each part and linking the entire system together in a whole harmoniously functioning organism. This energy system forms a microcosm of the universal energy patterns that run like templates throughout nature and the cosmos, from the galactic and solar systems down to the cellular, molecular, and atomic levels of existence. Containing multiple subsystems, such as organs, tissues, and cells, and contained within multiple supersystems, such as environmental, ecological, planetary, and solar systems, the human energy system shares the same basic elements and energies that constitute the entire universe, and human health depends entirely on the degree to which the energy system functions in resonant synchronicity with all its sub- and supersystems.

To continue functioning, all energy systems must achieve a balanced state of equilibrium between input and output. According to the Taoist paradigm of the Three Powers of Heaven, Earth, and Humanity, the human energy system stands midway between the forces of the cosmos (Heaven) and the forces of nature (Earth), assimilating energies from both sources and transforming them into the types of energy required by the human organism. Above, the human body acts as a superconductor for the subtle wave energies of Heaven constantly raining down on our heads from the sky, converting them into electromagnetic energy pulses that the human system can utilize. Below, the body extracts and assimilates the elemental energies of Earth contained in food, fluids, herbs, and air, transforming and refining them into the basic organic energies required by the human system. The more efficient the human system becomes at conducting and transducing the pure potent energies of the cosmos, such as light, color, and invisible rays, the less it must depend on grosser sources of energy such as food, herbs, and nutritional supplements. On the human balance sheet of income and expenditure, energy is always the bottom line.

Modern Western physics has clearly established a fact of life that traditional Eastern mystics discovered many millennia ago—that matter is nothing more nor less than condensed, highly organized energy. Einstein proposed this view half a century ago with his famous equation $E = mc^2$, but Western medicine has failed to realize the implications of this scientific fact for human health and medical care. "Science tells us that everything is energy and that matter is nothing more than energy in different form," explains energy therapist John Veltheim. "Our bodies are a composite of many different energy patterns and vibrations." As the "glue" that binds together all molecules, cells, tissues, and organs, the fuel that powers all vital functions, and the agent that executes the mind's commands, energy is by far the single most important constituent in the human system and the most vital factor in human health and longevity. It is the true "staff of life" and the bridge that links body and mind.

THE DYNAMICS OF YIN AND YANG

Human energy is an electromagnetic force that functions by virtue of its dynamic polarity. In Chinese tradition, this polarity, which manifests itself throughout the material universe, is called The Great Principle of Yin and Yang, and it explains the polar nature of all events and phenomena from the galactic and planetary macrocosms down to the organic, cellular, and molecular microcosms of the human energy system. Owing to the polarity of yin and yang, human energy, like all natural forces, is always moving, constantly transforming, ever active.

It is important to bear in mind that yin and yang are not two different types of energy, but rather opposite and complementary qualities of the same basic energies. The terms *yin* and *yang*, which first appeared in the *Book of Change (I-Ching)* around 1250 BCE, originally meant "the shady side of a hill" and "the sunny side of a hill" respectively, indicating that they are simply opposite sides of the same coin. Not only does this definition reflect the basic polar nature of yin and yang, it also indicates their mutually transmutable relationship, for as the sun (i.e., energy) moves across the sky, the shady side of the hill becomes sunny and the sunny side grows shady, just as water (yin) transforms into its own opposite element, steam (yang), when exposed to the Fire energy of heat. As the *I-Ching* states, "The interaction of yin and yang is called the Way [Tao], and the resulting creative process is called change." All creation and change are therefore prompted by the dynamic polarity of yin and yang, which are properties of active energy, not static matter.

Yin and yang manifest their complementary polarity in every aspect of the human system (see table 1). There are yin organs functionally coupled by energy with yang organs, "hot" energies and "cold" energies, expanding and contracting energies, "evil" (disease-causing) and "true" (healing) energies. The front of the body is yin relative to the back, which is yang; the external surface is yang vis-à-vis the yin interior; acid pH is yang while alkaline is yin; and so forth. Thus the essential nature of yin and yang is complementary polarity, their essential relationship is one of constant interaction and mutual

TABLE 1. Aspects of Yin-Yang Polarity

Aspects	Yin	Yang
UNIVERSAL MACROCOSM		
Celestial	Moon	Sun
Time	Midnight	Noon
Season	Winter, autumn	Summer, spring
Temperature	Cold, cool	Hot, warm
Light	Dark	Radiant
Composition	Hard, dense, heavy	Soft, porous, light
Form	Matter	Energy
Numbers	Even	Odd
Gender	Female	Male
Direction	Down	Up
Location	Below, inside, back	Above, outside, front
Activity	Formative, condensing	Transformative, expanding
HUMAN MICROCOSM		
Anatomy	Interior, lower torso and trunk, back, right side	Exterior, upper torso and head, front, left side
Vital organs	Liver, heart, spleen, lungs, kidneys	Gallbladder, small intestine, stomach, large intestine
System constituent	Essence (*jing*): Blood, fluids, tissues	Energy (*chee*): Heat, metabolic activity
Metabolism	Anabolism (tissue growth)	Catabolism (tissue breakdown)
Energy condition	Weak, empty, deficient, cold	Strong, full, excessive, hot
Life phases	Degeneration, death, development	Growth, birth, maturity
Psychic type	Contemplative, introverted, gentle	Active, extroverted, robust

transformation, and the dynamic balance between the two determines the state of health of the whole and of all its constituent parts.

Chinese philosophy cites five basic laws governing the ways in which the Great Principle of Yin and Yang functions in nature and throughout the cosmos, and Chinese medicine applies the same principles to the microcosmic universe within the human energy system.

1. All events and phenomena have two complementary polar aspects, called yin and yang, and this polarity is the basis of all organic structures and their functions.
2. Every yin-yang system contains myriad constituent subsystems and also is contained within myriad yin-yang supersystems.
3. Yin and yang mutually give rise to one another and are functionally dependent on one another. Their activities are always relative and their qualities complementary.
4. Yin and yang naturally balance and regulate each other. Their relative balance determines the equilibrium, stability, and functional viability of the whole human energy system and each of its organic subsystems.
5. Yin and yang are transmutable and mutually transform into each other. Their transformations initiate all creation, growth, change, and decline.

In the practice of Chinese medicine, the principle of yin and yang provides a convenient scale by which to gauge the overall equilibrium of the human energy system as well as the relative balance of all its constituent organ-energy subsystems. In diagnosis, it serves as a tool for determining the basic nature of specific ailments and monitoring their progression within the whole system. In therapy, it indicates the type of medical treatment required to rebalance ailing organ-energy systems and restore their synchronicity within the whole system. *Hot* and *cold, full* and *empty, external* and *internal, ascending* and *descending,* and many other terms used in traditional Chinese diagnosis and therapy are simply different ways of describing various manifestations of yin and yang polarity in different parts of the human system.

THE FIVE ELEMENTAL ENERGIES

The Five Elemental Energies (*wu hsing*), also translated as the Five Phases, are fundamental forces of nature created by the interplay of yin and yang on earth. An ancient Chinese treatise on energy states:

> By the transformation of yang and its union with yin, the Five Elemental Energies of Wood, Fire, Earth, Metal, and Water arise, each with its own specific nature according to its share of yin and yang. . . . The Five Elemental Energies combine and recombine in countless ways to create manifest existence. All things contain all Five Elemental Energies in various proportions.

As part of manifest nature on earth, the human system also evolved from various combinations of the Five Elemental Energies. *The Yellow Emperor's Classic of Internal Medicine* states, "It is a paradigm that applies equally to humans."

The activities, transformations, and cyclic phases mediated by the Five Elemental Energies in nature and in humans are all governed by a dynamic system of mutual checks and balances known as creative (*sheng*) and control (*keh*) cycles, or Mother/Son and Victor/Vanquished relationships. These complementary cycles automatically adjust the overall balance and functional harmony of the whole system according to the relative polarities of yin and yang in various interactions of the Five Elemental Energies. Whenever a condition of imbalance arises between two energies and their respective functions, the creative and control cycles compensate and correct the imbalance, restoring functional harmony to the whole system.

In the creative cycle, each energy generates and increases the one that follows, while in the control cycle, each energy subjugates and decreases the next one (fig. 3). Whenever a particular energy in the creative cycle flares up and exerts an excessively stimulating influence over the following energy, the control cycle automatically counteracts that excess influence by sugjugating the flaring energy with its controlling element. If this natural balancing mechanism fails to function because of obstructions or other problems in the human energy system, the uncompensated imbalance of energies will soon manifest somatically and give rise to physiological disease, in which case a physician must step in to correct the problem with herbs, acupuncture, and/or other therapies that rebalance the human energy system. For example, an overactive heart (Fire) will eventually overstimulate the spleen (Earth) by virtue of the creative relationship of Fire to Earth, and if this condition of imbalance continues uncorrected, serious digestive problems might occur. The Chinese physician may correct this condition in two ways: either directly sedate the heart's Fire to take pressure off the spleen's Earth, or else stimulate the kidneys' Water to subjugate the heart's Fire through the control cycle of Water over Fire, thereby also relieving the spleen's Earth energy of excess Fire influence. In Chinese medicine, human health always boils down to the basic balance and harmony of energies within the system.

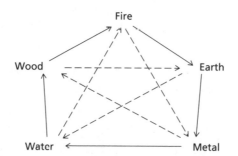

Figure 3. The creative cycle (solid lines) and control cycle (dotted lines) of the Five Elemental Energies of nature.

Chinese medicine defines the vital organs not in terms of their forms, locations, and biochemical constituents, but rather in terms of the energies that govern them and the vital functions they operate within the whole system. Those organ energies and their functions are viewed in terms of the polar balance between yin and yang and the cyclic harmony among the Five Elemental Energies. The universal laws governing the activities of yin and yang and the Five Elemental Energies in nature thus form a master template by which the physician may understand the internal workings of the human system and trace the root imbalances of energy responsible for particular symptoms of physiological disease. These laws and the organic relationships they control also provide the physician with a vehicle for regulating the patient's energies to restore balance and harmony to the whole system, thereby eliminating the root causes of disease in the body.

The Five Elemental Energies permeate every realm of nature and function ceaselessly on all three levels of human existence—body (*jing*), energy (*chee*), and mind (*shen*), the Three Treasures of life. In the physical body, they manage the functions and determine the conditions of all the vital organs, glands and tissues. In the energy system, or "auric body," they manifest as emotions and feelings and mediate the myriad energy transformations within the system and between the system and the external environment. On the level of mind, the Five Energies are related to various mental faculties such as will, intuition, and creativity. Chinese medicine also distinguishes various constitutional energy types based on which of these five forces prevails in an individual's system, such as the hot, hyperactive Fire constitution, the expansive and creative Wood type, the cool, conserving Water system, and so forth. These designations may be determined according to various external signs, such as complexion, physique, tone of hair, skin, and nails, color and texture of tongue, and so forth, and they assist the physician in diagnosis as well as therapy.

Each human being is endowed by nature and genetics with various different proportions and relative strengths of the Five Elemental Energies. Any inherent deficiencies and imbalances may be supplemented and replenished during the course of life by tapping various external sources of these energies, such as food, herbs, aromas, sunlight, atmospheric elements, and so on. Energy from such external sources may be cultivated and assimilated either by personal practices such as diet, exercise, sexual yoga, *chee-gung*, and meditation, or else by holistic medical therapies like herbs, acupuncture, massage, and so forth. In each case, a specific external energy is brought into the system by virtue of its resonance or "natural affinity" (*gui jing*) with a particular internal organ-energy, with one of the Five Elemental Energies serving as a common denominator between the external source and the internal organ. Sweet herbs, for example, replenish spleen and stomach energy, because sweet is an Earth-energy flavor while the spleen and stomach are Earth-energy organs. By the same principle, sour herbs and foods (Wood energy) boost liver and gallbladder functions (Wood organs), pungent (Metal) flavors influence the lungs and large intestine (Metal organs), and so forth. Acupuncture works by directly modulating the flow and potential of the various internal organ-energies running through the meridian network, increasing or decreasing their strength according to the physician's purposes. Therefore, all Chinese therapies are basically methods of energy transfer and energy control achieved by establishing resonance between various external sources of healing energy and the internal organ-energies for which those particular sources have natural affinities. The goal of all these therapies is to restore natural balance and harmony within the human energy system and establish synchronicity between the whole system and the energy cycles of nature and the cosmos.

Ultimately, all matter is created and controlled by the Five Elemental Energies, and eventually all matter returns to these energies in their pure primordial form as colored rays of light. According to

Taoist as well as Buddhist thought, the ultimate fundamental nature of mind and all reality is the radiant luminosity of primordial Clear Light. From the Clear Light of primordial spirit, which is eternal and infinite, the mind refracts the five colored rays and uses them to condense and organize the free self-existent energy of the universe into the various forms of matter and organic energy that compose our physical bodies and material world. Yellow rays of light possess the unique capacity to organize the elemental energy of Earth, which constitutes the "meat and bones" of our bodies as well as the planet we inhabit. Red controls the elemental energy of Fire, which brings heat to the earth and warmth to our bodies. Water energy creates the blood and other fluids in our bodies and gives rise to the rivers, lakes, and oceans of the earth, and so forth. During the course of life, the Five Elemental Energies flow through our systems, managing their respective tissues and functions and drawing on external sources for replenishment and balance. But when we die, our spirits withdraw these energies from our dying bodies one by one, beginning with Earth, then Water, in consecutive order, and as each energy is transformed back into the pure primordial light from which it sprang, the corresponding organs and energies of the body cease to function, until the body is dead and all its constituent energies have been reabsorbed into the original Clear Light of primordial spirit, ready to be projected into whatever realm of existence and form of life come next. The Chinese refer to this process of energy reintegration at death as Returning to the Source, and it marks the boundary where medical science ends and spiritual practice begins.

The major organs, colors, sounds, flavors, emotions, seasons, and other manifest qualities of nature are associated with each of the Five Elemental Energies in Chinese medicine and other Taoist disciplines (see table 2). Readers may consult this chart to determine their own individual energy types, based on the predilections listed, and to adjust their personal habits and lifestyles for better balance and harmony. Note that Fire governs an extra set of paired organs

TABLE 2. The Five Elemental Energies and Their Macrocosmic and Microcosmic Associations

Category	Wood	Fire	Earth	Metal	Water
UNIVERSAL MACROCOSM					
Color	Green	Red	Yellow	White	Black
Flavor	Sour	Bitter	Sweet	Pungent	Salty
Climate	Windy	Hot	Damp	Dry	Cold
Hours	3–7 A.M.	9 A.M.–1 P.M.	1–3, 7–9 A.M. 1–3, 7–9 P.M.	3–7 P.M.	9 P.M.–1 A.M.
Development phase	Sprouting, growing	Blooming, fruiting	Ripening, harvesting	Withering, decaying	Dormancy, storage
Direction	East	South	Center	West	North
Season	Spring	Summer	Late summer	Autumn	Winter
Activity	Generates	Expands	Stabilizes	Contracts	Conserves
HUMAN MICROCOSM					
Organ Yin	Liver	Heart, pericardium	Spleen	Lungs	Kidneys
Yang	Gallbladder	Small intestine, Triple Burner	Stomach	Large intestine	Bladder
Vital function	Nervous system	Blood, endocrine	Digestion, lymph, muscle	Respiration, skin	Urinary, reproductive
Bodily secretions	Tears	Sweat	Saliva	Mucus	Urine, sexual fluids
Emotion	Anger	Joy	Obsession	Grief	Fear
External apertures	Eyes	Tongue, throat	Lips, mouth	Nose	Ears
Life cycle	Infancy	Youth	Maturity	Old age	Death
Healing sound	Hsü	Her	Hoo	Shee	Chway
Tissue	Ligaments, nerves, nails	Blood vessels	Fat, muscle	Skin, hair	Bones, marrow, brain
PSYCHIC AND PERSONALITY TRAITS					
Energy type	Expanding	Fusing	Moderating	Condensing	Conserving
Ability	Initiative	Communication	Negotiation	Discrimination	Imagination
Mental preoccupation	Work	Stimulation	Detail	Ritual	Secret, mystery
Obsessions	Answers, choices, goals	Pleasure, desire, love, divinity	Manipulation, loyalties, security	Perfection, order, standards	Mysteries, death, visions, facts
Tendencies	Risk, busy work	Excitement, contact	Comfort, company	Follow orders, make judgments	Solitude, isolation
Emotional need	Arousal	Being in love	Being needed	Being right	Being protected
Psychic fear	Helplessness	Isolation	Confusion	Corruption	Extinction
Virtue	Benevolence	Propriety	Faith	Rectitude	Wisdom
Emotional weakness	Depression	Instability	Obsession	Anguish	Fear

not recognized in Western medicine—the pericardium and Triple Burner. The former is associated with cardiac function and protects the heart from aberrant energies, while the latter is involved with the three basic functions of ingestion, digestion, and excretion. Neither are organs in the strict sense of Western anatomy, and the functions of both are governed by Fire energy, which is all that need concern us here.

TYPES OF HUMAN ENERGY

Chinese medicine distinguishes two fundamental forms of energy in the human system: prenatal, or primordial (*hsien-tien*); and postnatal, or temporal (*hou-tien*), also known as Water and Fire. Prenatal energy is the basic vital force with which we are endowed at birth; it is inherited from the genetic plasma of our parents, and it is stored in the sexual glands and reproductive cells. Usually referred to as *yuan-chee* (primordial energy), it constitutes a sort of "bio-battery" from which we can draw energy when external sources such as food and air are insufficient, but each of us is born with a limited supply, and it cannot be replaced. Therefore, if we burn up all our reserve *yuan-chee* because of negligent health habits and careless lifestyles, our bodies will rapidly deteriorate, and lifespan is shortened.

Postnatal or Fire energy is the energy we assimilate from external sources through digestion and respiration and transform into human energy. It constitutes the basic fuel of life and takes various different functional forms in the human system. The type of energy specifically required by the human system is called True Energy (*jeng-chee*), and it is produced in the bloodstream from the fusion of the energy extracted from food by the stomach, spleen, and pancreas, and the energy extracted from air by the lungs. True Energy then takes two basic forms in the human system, depending on function: one is called nourishing energy (*ying-chee*) and the other is guardian energy (*wei-chee*). Nourishing energy travels within the blood vessels and energy meridians, where it works with the Five Elemental Energies of the organ systems and provides the fuel for the body's various vital processes. Guardian energy runs outside the bloodstream and meridians, along the body's surface, just below the skin, forming an aura of protective energy that prevents aberrant external energies from invading the human system and causing disease.

All these various types of energy are coordinated by the human system to sustain the health and functional integrity of the whole body and all its parts. These energies are constantly transformed and transferred throughout the system to meet the body's needs and to compensate for shifting conditions in the environment, and the overall balance and functional harmony among them determines the state of one's physical and mental health. Only when the human system achieves a stable and balanced state of physical and mental health can it produce and utilize the subtlest of all human energies—*ling-chee*, or spirit energy—which is transformed within the system from ordinary energies through the internal alchemy (*nei-gung*) of meditation and *chee-gung* practice. This pure, highly refined energy enhances awareness and boosts mental powers; it is also the basic component of the so-called spiritual embryo of enlightened awareness cultivated by advanced spiritual adepts, who use it as a vehicle for carrying consciousness beyond the body at death. Known in Tibetan yoga as the Rainbow Body, this subtle body of pure primordial light is the ultimate goal of those who practice the most advanced stages of Taoist and Tibetan Buddhist meditation. Although this aspect of human energy lies beyond the scope of medical science, which concerns itself only with life before death, not after, it is mentioned here to give the reader a glimpse of how the basic energies involved in physical health are related in Chinese medicine to the higher goals of spiritual practice.

THE HUMAN ENERGY NETWORK

Chinese medicine recognizes three circulatory networks in the human system: the nerves, blood vessels, and energy meridians.

Western medicine acknowledges only the first two, but Chinese medicine regards the third to be by far the most important. *The Yellow Emperor's Classic of Internal Medicine* states, "Energy commands blood; where energy goes, blood follows." This means that blood circulates only in tissues where energy is already flowing freely, and that the cause of insufficient blood circulation is a blockage in the energy meridians. The same principle applies to the nervous system, and that is why, in Chinese medicine, both blood circulation and nervous system disorders can be corrected by acupuncture and other therapies that stimulate and balance the flow of energy through the meridian network, which forms an invisible template that both the blood and nervous systems follow. All three circulatory systems must be properly balanced and functioning in synchronicity to sustain health, but it is the meridian network and its subtle energies that must be manipulated and restored to correct problems in all three systems. So once again we note the primacy of energy in the Chinese approach to human health.

The Chinese have known about the invisible human energy network for at least five thousand years. They discovered that human energy flows through the body through a complex grid of major channels (*mai*), organ meridians (*jing*), and minor capillaries (*luo*), along which they also found a series of sensitive energy points (*hsueh*) that function as transformers and relay terminals for human energy. These points, each of which has specific effects on specific organs, tissues, and related energies, are the basis of acupuncture, moxibustion, and acupressure therapies.

The most powerful channels in the human energy network, the Eight Extraordinary Channels (*chi jing ba mai*), serve as reservoirs of energy for the entire system and may be activated and replenished by *chee-gung*, meditation, and other practices. The most important of these eight are called the Governing and Conception Channels, which form what is known as the Microcosmic Orbit, from which the entire system draws energy. Next come the twelve meridians associated with the twelve vital organ-energy systems. These meridians run like rivers throughout the system, irrigating organs, glands, and tissues with nourishing energy and managing their respective vital functions. These meridians circulate energy to the major organ systems in a specific order (fig. 4). Branching out from the eight major channels and twelve organ meridians are countless smaller capillaries, forming a finely woven web that feeds energy to every cell in the body.

The human energy network serves many purposes. It regulates blood circulation and blood pressure, maintains the body's external shell of guardian energy, mediates the nervous system, distributes

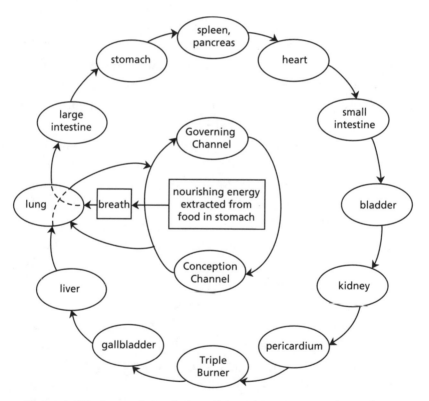

Figure 4. The internal circulation of nourishing energy to the vital organ-energy systems, with the Governing and Conception Channels as reservoirs.

nourishing energy throughout the system, controls body heat, fuels metabolism, forms all functional links between body and mind, and much more. In Chinese medicine, all physiological pathology, as well as mental and emotional problems, are seen as symptomatic reflections of critical imbalances or malfunctions within the human energy network, which also provides the primary vehicle through which the physician may cure the patient's ailments.

THE HUMAN ENERGY FIELD

So far, we have discussed the various *forms* of energy in the human system and how they *function* and circulate, but of equal importance to health is the strength and polarity of the *field* in which human energy operates and from which it draws its power. All electromagnetic energies, including those of the human system, create an electromagnetic field. The human energy field is composed of many constituent subfields created by the energies of various component organs, tissues, and individual cells, and is also part of various superfields in which it operates, such as groups, dwellings, ecosystems, geographic regions, and the electromagnetic field of the planet itself. All these systems must resonate in synchronicity to prevent the imbalances and aberrations in energy that cause disease and degeneration. In *Pranayama: The Yoga of Breathing*, Andre van Lysebeth writes:

> The longevity of civilized man depends to a very high degree on the continual presence of a sufficiently powerful electric field. . . . A great many so-called 'modern illnesses' [e.g., cancer, AIDS] can be traced to the absence or considerable reduction in intensity of the natural electric fields in big towns. Human beings who are forced to live in buildings or rooms with metal frames and which therefore have the physical properties of a Faraday cage, from which any electric field is excluded, tire and are exhausted quickly.

Richard Broeringmeyer, publisher of *Bio-Energy Health Newsletter*, puts it like this: "Life is not possible without electromagnetic fields, and optimum health is not possible if the electromagnetic fields are out of balance for long periods of time." The human body generates an electromagnetic field that extends about 1 meter outward, with one pole at the head and the other at the perineum. Any force that blocks or unbalances the natural human energy field is a potential cause of disease. That is why many Chinese doctors refuse to treat patients who insist on wearing quartz crystal watches: the high-frequency oscillations from the crystal interfere with human energy pulses (which are particularly sensitive on the wrists) and distort the human energy field, thereby obstructing all therapies that deal with the human energy system, as Chinese therapies do.

The human energy field is directy influenced by, and can draw energy from, all sorts of other natural electromagnetic fields, such as those of the sun, moon, planets, and stars, as well as the earth's own field, and it can also be polluted by negative fields created by electric power lines and transformers, electrical appliances, broadcasting towers, metal-frame construction, microwave radiation, and other artificial sources. In diagnosing and treating human disease, it is therefore just as important to consider the effects of exposure to harmful external energy fields as it is to trace imbalances in internal energies. If your headaches are caused by sleeping in a room that exposes your system to the electromagnetic field created by a nearby electric power transformer or household appliance, it will not do you much good to take acupuncture, herbs, or any other therapy for headaches unless you first eliminate the root source of the problem by sleeping in a different room or removing the offending source of electromagnetic pollution from your home.

The human energy field is what Gabriel Cousens, author of *Spiritual Nutrition and the Rainbow Diet*, calls a Subtle Organizing Energy Field (SOEF). Such fields, which are present in all forms of life, organize all the energies and elements required to maintain organic life forms. In humans, SOEFs arrange the energies and elements of the human system according to the master template patterns contained in DNA, which choreographs all the body's vital functions in the harmonious symphony of life. By virtue of their power to organize random energies into patterned forms, SOEFs work against the life-threatening influence of the second law of thermodynamics, or entropy, which causes the eventual dissolution of all composite systems in the universe. As long as the human energy system and its SOEF remain balanced and fully charged with polar energy, they will automatically repair all damage to the physical organism, maintain all vital functions, and resist the decaying force of entropy.

Whenever the human energy field is invaded by aberrant internal or external energies or exposed to harmful artificial energy fields, the entire system is thrown off balance and loses its functional harmony. If this situation of imbalance is not promptly corrected, physiological pathology and abnormal mental and emotional symptoms will soon follow. Simply suppressing the physical and mental symptoms of disease to provide quick relief, as is the practice in Western allopathic medicine, will never effect a lasting cure as long as the underlying energy imbalances that caused the symptoms are allowed to remain. When suppressive allopathic medication is applied, the external symptoms of internal energy imbalance continue to shift, transform, and manifest elsewhere in the body, often leading the allopathic doctor to diagnose a different disease and apply a different drug to treat the "new" symptom, whereas the Chinese doctor sees the new symptom as just another manifestation of the same old problem, a clear indication that the root cause in the energy system has not been successfully corrected. In Chinese medicine, the only true cure for all disease, dysfunction, and degeneration in the human body is to restore balance to unbalanced energies and functional harmony to dysfunctional systems, and to reestablish synchronicity among all the sub- and supersystems that influence the human energy field.

CHAKRAS AND SUBTLE ENERGY BODIES

The dynamic force field enveloping the human energy system is actually composed of seven subtle energy "bodies," each of them managed by one of the seven subtle energy centers known as chakras, which radiate the wave frequency of specific colors and are functionally associated with specific glands and nerve networks (fig. 5). The colors, which the mind refracts like a prism from the Clear Light of primordial spirit, are pure forms of universal free energy, and each one regulates specific aspects of the human energy system. The subtle energy bodies, also known as auras, extend outward from the physical body as luminous energy fields, with the densest ones closest to the physical surface and the subtlest ones radiating far beyond.

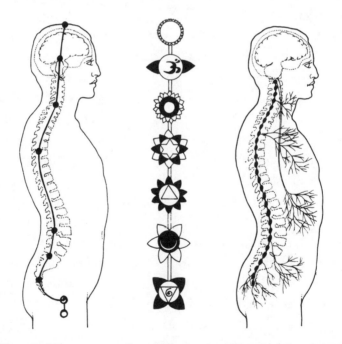

Figure 5. The correspondence between the energy centers of Taoist internal alchemy, the chakras of Indian yoga, and the nerve centers of Western anatomy.

The chakras, known in Taoist internal alchemy as elixir fields (*dan-tien*), function as two-way transformers: they "step down" and transduce the cosmic energies entering our systems from the sky into forms and frequencies that can be utilized by the body; and they "step up" and refine the lower energies of earth into forms and frequencies that can be used by the mind. The upper three chakras are therefore involved mostly with higher spiritual energies, whereas the three lower ones deal mostly with the coarser physiological energies of food, sex, and other earthbound forces. The center heart chakra balances the two and controls them with human consciousness.

Invisible cosmic energies are constantly entering our systems through the crown (pineal) chakra, which immediately transfers them down to the brow (pituitary) chakra, where they are refracted into the seven colored rays. These are, in descending order, violet, indigo, sky blue, green, yellow, orange, and red. When this colored light energy reaches the heart (thymus) chakra, it is transformed into Fire (heat) energy, a denser form of energy utilized by the lower chakras. At the root (genital) chakra, the energy is further condensed into a denser form that Jack Schwartz, author of *Human Energy Systems*, refers to as molasses. When this type of energy, which also enters the body from the earth through the perineum, rises back up through the chakra system, it is once again transformed into progressively subtler forms, until it reaches the crown again as the pure cosmic light energy of primordial spirit. The energy centers and the transformations they mediate are important elements in Taoist internal alchemy practices.

Because the upper three centers (throat, brow, crown) are involved mainly with the mental and spiritual processes of meditation, or Heaven, Chinese medicine deals primarily with the three lower centers (root, navel, solar plexus), which regulate the functions of the physical body and its vital organs, or Earth. In this paradigm, the heart center represents the power of Humanity, whose consciousness stands between and balances the powers of Heaven above and Earth below to sustain the overall welfare of the whole system, spiritual as well as physical. In the Chinese system of health care, the physician deals directly with the Earth energies of the three lower centers, and it remains up to the individual to cultivate the higher spiritual energies of Heaven under the guidance of a qualified spiritual master. Optimum health and longevity can be achieved when all the Three Powers (*san tsai*) of Heaven, Earth, and Humanity are properly cultivated and harmoniously integrated in the human system.

THE BODY AS COSMIC SUPERCONDUCTOR AND ENERGY TRANSFORMER

Certain human tissues, particularly the bones, ligaments, and other connective tissues, have a distinctive crystalline structure with piezo-electric properties, which means that they, like all crystals, generate an electromagnetic field pulse whenever physically stimulated or stressed. As crystal structures, bones especially have the unique capacity to transduce vibrational wave energy such as light, sound, and physical palpation into electromagnetic energy pulses that can be assimilated and utilized by the human energy system. This explains, for example, how the sound energy of mantra and music may be used to energize and heal the human system. The body's crystalline structures absorb the vibrations and convert them into electromagnetic energy signals that directly influence the human energy system. Perhaps this is one reason that singers and dancers, barring the self-destructive behavior to which many are so prone, tend to live longer lives and enjoy more robust health than other people. The rhythmic pulses of song and dance generate healing frequencies in their bones and other crystalline tissues, which then broadcast healing electromagnetic pulses to the rest of the body, particularly organs and glands.

Conversely, it has been scientifically shown that electromagnetic pulses can affect and alter the physical structure of crystals, such as bone and other human tissues, which explains how acupuncture can heal tissues by modulating electromagnetic signals in the meridian network. It also explains why pulsed electromagnetic fields can be used to stimulate the healing of broken bones and activate secretions of hormones and neurochemicals.

Because the crystalline structures of human tissues are so sensitive to even the subtlest changes in the ambient electromagnetic fields to which they are exposed, it should be obvious that the abnormal artificial electromagnetic fields produced by power lines, transformers, broadcasting towers, radar installations, and electrical appliances have highly deleterious effects on the human body. Evidence suggests that these artificial electromagnetic fields, which did not exist on earth prior to the twentieth century, are deeply involved as contributing factors in many of the mortal maladies that plague modern humanity, such as cancer and AIDS.*

Besides bones and other solid crystalline tissues, the human body is packed with liquid crystal structures such as blood, lymph, hormones, and intercellular fluids. These also have piezoelectric properties, constantly converting incoming vibratory wave energy into electromagnetic fields and energy pulses that stimulate and heal the human system. Certain bodily fluids, such as cell salts, also have the capacity to store and transfer energy in the form of electrically charged ions. All these crystal structures form a series of interpenetrating, oscillating energy fields and subfields, all of which must resonate in synchronicity throughout the whole system to sustain health and vitality.

As can be plainly seen from the above discussion, the body's molecular and energy structures are inseparably related, with the crystalline structures of tissues transforming and transferring energies, and the energies managing the formation and dissolution of molecules, cells, and tissues. The important point to remember is that the invis-

---

*See S. Becker, *Cross Currents* (Los Angeles: Jeremy Tarcher, 1990).

ible energies associated with cells, tissues, and organs constitute the dynamic force of human life and are always the primary factors in health and disease, whereas the physical tissues are simply material shells in which the vital energies of human life function. Disease and degeneration in the physical body always indicate serious imbalances and functional disorders in the human energy system and can therefore be successfully treated only with therapies that restore balance and harmony to the whole energy system and all its constituent organ subsystems.

Each and every organ-energy system and cellular subsystem in the body has its own unique electromagnetic frequency. Whenever the energy of a particular system is suppressed, overstimulated, chilled, heated, dampened, or otherwise distorted by aberrant energies and abnormal energy fields, the related organs and tissues suffer physiological damage and begin to malfunction, causing the whole system to feel a sense of "dis-ease." By manipulating the specific frequencies of ailing organ-energies with acupuncture, herbs, *chee-gung*, sound, light, massage, and other holistic energy therapies, the physician rebalances those energies and restores their synchronicity with the whole system. Once restored, these energies immediately go to work reorganizing the molecules, rebuilding the cells, and restoring the functions of the diseased organs and tissues, and all physical as well as mental symptoms of disease disappear. No doctor can actually heal a damaged or diseased body. The best he or she can do is to restore the energy balance and functional harmony on which human health depends, so that the system can heal itself.

Chinese medicine has always stressed the vital importance of bones and bodily fluids in human health. These tissues function like antennae and transducers, picking up subtle energy vibrations from Heaven (stars, planets, and the cosmos) and from Earth (the forces of nature) and transforming them into the electromagnetic field energy of "Humanity." They broadcast these healing electromagnetic pulses to organs and glands throughout the system, based on the resonance or natural affinity between the original energy sources and specific parts of the body. This is also one reason why it is so important to keep your bones properly aligned, and why therapeutic Chinese exercises focus so much on loosening, relaxing, and aligning bones and joints, stretching and toning ligaments and tendons, and stimulating circulation of blood, bile, lymph, and other crystalline bodily fluids.

The old adage, "you can feel it in your bones," is literally true for those who have developed keen sensitivity to the energy pulses generated in their skeletal structures when listening, for example, to moving music or other mellifluous sounds, or whenever they have moving thoughts and emotions, or are exposed to strong external energy vibrations, all of which create powerful waves of energy that are immediately picked up and transformed into electromagnetic pulses by the bones.

From the solid, innermost skeletal core of the physical body all the way out to the subtlest, outermost ring of the finest auric energy body, the human energy system consists of an overlapping series of interdependent, oscillating energy fields that draw energy into the human system from many different sources, transforming it into the True Energy of the human system and organizing it to sustain the molecules, cells, tissues, and organs of the physical body. From beginning to end, energy is always the key factor in all the equations of human health, the vehicle for healing, the basis of all therapies, the bridge between physical and mental phenomena, and the medium through which mind exerts ultimate control over matter. In the human system, energy is the most basic component and fundamental fact of life, the organizing force without which the elemental building blocks of air, water, and nutrition remain inert and lifeless.

3

The Causes of Disease

BASICALLY, THE MAIN CAUSE of disease is "bad weather," not germs. As Harriet Beinfield and Efrem Korngold put it in *Between Heaven and Earth: A Guide to Traditional Chinese Medicine*, "Whenever specific 'weather' starts to dominate the body milieu, it can become a pathogenic stress. This may be both the source and outcome, the root and fruit, of imbalance." Other than obvious physical trauma such as gunshot wounds or car accidents, the overwhelming majority of human health problems are caused by aberrant energies that knock the human energy system off balance, creating the sort of abnormal "climate" inside the body that permits germs and other pathogens to enter the system. It is the state of the human energy system, particularly the immune response, that determines whether the body become vulnerable or remains resistant to invasion by germs. Deadly germs and parasites are *always* present inside and outside the human body, which means that our systems are *always* exposed to them. For example, nearly 80 percent of all humans carry the pneumonia bacillus in their lungs. But the germs remain dormant and benign rather than a threat to human health as long as "favorable winds" prevail in the human energy system and the immune response remains strong. When normal energy balance is

46

upset by malnutrition, toxic blood, polluted tissues, abnormal energy fields, and other disruptive factors, the immune response is impaired, and the ever-present germs, fungi, and parasites in our internal and external environments have a field day invading and colonizing our systems. If germs themselves were the actual *cause* of disease, we would all be dead within minutes of being born into this toxic, germ-infested world.

In Chinese medicine, the root cause of most types of disease and degeneration is traced to a critical imbalance in various organ-energies of the body, and to the overall functional disharmony of the whole system that invariably results from organic imbalance. Owing to the interdependence of the Three Treasures of body, energy, and mind, energy imbalance *always* manifests in the body as physical disease and discomfort and in the mind as mental and emotional malaise. The corollary to this principle is that all symptoms of physical as well as mental and emotional disease can *always* be tracked back to specific imbalances and functional disharmony in the energy system. The root causes of disease always occur first in the invisible web of the human energy system, and the primary causative factors are aberrant energies, not microbes. By the time symptoms appear in the body or mind, the root causes have already become so entrenched in the energy system that they have critically impaired the immune response and inhibited other vital functions, thereby establishing the abnormal conditions that allow disease and degeneration to occur on the physical plane. By predicting the "weather" in the human energy system, the Chinese physician is able to take preventive measures to maintain optimum balance and functional harmony within the system, eliminating the conditions of heat, cold, damp, dryness, and other energy imbalances that give rise to the physical and mental symptoms of disease.

Owing to modern technology and contemporary urban lifestyles, the internal and external energies that decisively influence human health and longevity are far more complex and potentially harmful today than they ever were in ancient times. The aberrant environmental and atmospheric energies of nature known in traditional Chinese medicine as the Six Evils, such as heat, cold, damp, dryness, and so forth, have now been eclipsed in magnitude and danger by the "dry-heat" of central heating, the "dry-cold" of air conditioning, the "evil winds" of microwave radiation and artificial electromagnetic fields, the internal "damp-heat" of white sugar, alcohol, and chemical drugs, and other artificial industrial sources of abnormal energies that play havoc with the natural balance and patterns of human energies. The same goes for the internal landscape of mental and emotional energies. In traditional times, the disruptive energies of the Seven Emotions (grief, anger, fear, and so forth) were regarded as the primary internal causes of disease, but today the impact of these disturbing emotions has been greatly amplified and complicated by stress, neurosis, psychosis, pananoia, *angst*, and other debilitating mental and emotional energies generated in response to the pace and pressure of modern urban lifestyles.

Nevertheless, regardless of how lethal and complex the energy factors influencing human health today have become, it is still the balance between positive and negative, healing and harmful, yin and yang energies, and the overall harmony of the whole system that determine whether those factors remain benign or become malignant. If imbalances in the human energy system can be detected and corrected before they cause serious physical or mental symptoms, disease and degeneration can be prevented and life prolonged, and this remains the basic approach of traditional Chinese medicine to human health and healing in the modern age.

Modern Western medicine is based on Pasteur's germ theory of disease, also known as the single-agent theory, whereby every known disease is diagnosed as being caused by a specific pathogen found in the diseased tissues, then treated with chemical agents that destroy that specific pathogen. When the pathogen is no longer found in the body, the patient is declared cured and the medication is withdrawn.

This theory fails to explain the cause of cancer, arthritis, osteoporosis, arteriosclerosis, and many other degenerative conditions unrelated to germs, nor does it really even explain the nature of infectious diseases associated with germs, because it does not explain why under precisely the same conditions of exposure to exactly the same germs, some people catch the disease and others do not.

Let us use the analogy of garbage and flies to illustrate this point. Garbage always attracts flies, but that certainly does not mean that flies *cause* garbage. In fact, once the flies lay their eggs in the garbage, maggots appear. The garbage itself causes more flies! Using pesticide to kill the flies will not get rid of the garbage, and as soon as the pesticide wears off, more flies will come and colonize the same garbage. If you clean up the garbage, however, the flies will disappear all by themselves, for flies cannot live and breed in a clean, antiseptic environment, any more than germs can live in normal, healthy tissues.

Precisely the same principle applies to the germs that appear in toxic human tissues. Germs do not *cause* the toxicity and pathology of diseased tissues; they are *attracted* to those tissues by toxic conditions, and by the resulting lack of immune factors there. Killing those germs does nothing whatsoever to correct the tissue toxicity and immune deficiency that host them; on the contrary, the chemical drugs, radiation, and surgery favored by modern Western medicine only further aggravate tissue toxicity and further impair the immune response, paving the way for even more severe relapses later. The bottom line is this: *Pathogenic germs can live and breed only in abnormal conditions of extreme tissue toxicity and critically impaired immune response, not in normal, healthy tissues guarded by a strong immune system.* It is as simple as that.

Pathogenic germs are living organisms that require very specific conditions of temperature, humidity, pH, and other environmental factors to survive. Vintners and bakers are aware of this fact, and they must maintain precisely the right "climate" in their fermenting breads and wines to produce palatable products. Pasteur himself was well aware of the primacy of milieu over microbe, and his journals are full of references to specific conditions of internal climate that predispose tissues to infection by specific germs. Unfortunately, this aspect of Pasteur's work has been swept under the carpet by the modern medical industry, which has instead latched onto his highly tentative germ theory and has been waging "germ warfare" against diseased human bodies ever since, often with adverse effects for human health and longevity, not least of which has been the ominous appearance of mutant strains of pneumonia, malaria, tuberculosis, and other germs that are totally resistant to all drugs. Witnesses who were present at his deathbed say that Pasteur finally saw the light shortly before he died and recanted his germ theory of disease. "The microbe is nothing!" he declared. "The terrain is all!" Today, when many microbes have grown resistant to all drugs, the terrain has become more important than ever before in protecting human health.

It is the preexisting condition of the internal terrain in the human body that determines whether tissues will host or resist microbes and other pathogens, not the microbe itself. Long before Pasteur's dubious germ theory became canonized by modern Western medicine, the eighteenth-century cellular pathologist Rudolf Virchow wrote, "If I could live my life over again, I would devote it to proving that germs seek their *natural habitat—diseased tissue*—rather than being the cause of diseased tissue" (author's italics). Holistic healer Henry Bieler, author of *Food Is Your Best Medicine*, agrees. "The primary cause of disease is not germs," he writes. "Rather, I believe that disease is caused by a toxemia which results in cellular impairment and breakdown, thus paving the way for the multiplication and onslaught of germs." Yet despite such words of wisdom from within its own ranks, the entire Western medical and pharmaceutical industry, the most profitable industry in America today, remains firmly rooted in the single-agent germ theory that Pasteur himself ultimately rejected. Consequently, instead of cleaning up the internal garbage and tissue toxemia that paves the way for the onslaught of germs, Western medicine continues to escalate its chemical and surgical blitzkrieg against germs, using a slash and burn policy that lays further waste to the internal human terrain and permits even more virulent pathogens to enter the system.

In traditional Chinese medicine, the major external causes of disease are aberrant environmental and atmospheric energies known as the Six Evils (*liu shieh*): these are wind, heat, damp, dryness, cold, and fire. These noxious energies have debilitating influences on the human energy system, creating the conditions of imbalance and disharmony that permit disease to take root and create somatic and/or psychic symptoms. Traditionally associated with the Five Elemental Energies and their corresponding organs, seasons, colors, and other related factors (table 3), the five "evil" energies of wind, cold, heat,

TABLE 3. The Six Evils and Their Elemental Associations

Evil	Element	Season	Organs	Emotions	Effects
Wind	Wood	Spring	Liver, gall bladder	Anger	Scatters, upsets, disperses
Heat	Fire	Summer	Heart, small intestine	Joy	Accelerates, ascends, activates, warms
Damp	Earth	Late summer	Spleen, stomach	Worry	Sinks, accumulates, condenses, stagnates
Dryness	Metal	Autumn	Lungs, large intestine	Anxiety, grief	Shrinks, dehydrates, astringent
Cold	Water	Winter	Kidneys, bladder	Fear, fright	Chills, depresses, depletes, exhausts
Fire	Prolonged exposure to extreme conditions of any of the above gives rise to Fire, which intensifies symptoms and "burns out" the affected organs and tissues.				

damp, and dryness take even more aggressive form because of artificial external sources of aberrant energies, such as air conditioning and central heating, industrial and automobile pollution, microwaves and power lines, and processed foods and drugs. The sixth evil, fire, develops as a result of prolonged exposure to extreme conditions of any of the other five; left uncorrected, the conditions of imbalance caused by the other five evils grow steadily worse and eventually "burn out" the affected tissues and organs, hence the term *fire*. The Six Evils usually invade the human system in various combinations, such as dry-wind, cold-wind, hot-damp, cold-damp, and so forth, and each combination harms specific human energies and their related organs and tissues.

The primary internal causes of disease in Chinese medicine are called the Seven Emotions (*chi ching*), the unbridled waves of wild energy that stampede through the whole system as a result of extreme emotional reactions to external events. Because of the mental and physical disturbance it causes, emotion is also known in Taoist alchemy as the Chief Hooligan, while the five senses through which emotional reactions are provoked are called the Five Thieves, because they steal energy and awareness away from spirit and squander them instead on petty sensory distractions.

Emotions are direct internal responses by the human energy system to external stimuli perceived through the sensory channels. The essential nature of emotion and its role in human health are best understood when emotion is viewed as energy-in-motion (e-motion), rather than as the strictly psychological phenomenon perceived in Western medicine. Psychological factors are involved for only a brief instant in emotional response, at the moment when the mind reacts to incoming sensory signals in positive terms of attraction or negative terms of aversion, depending on personal bias. The same external event may provoke joy in one person, anger in another, and grief in yet a third, with very different psychological overtones, but in all three cases the energies unleashed by emotional response run rampant through the system, disrupting the delicate organic balance of the body's internal energies and impairing vital functions, particularly the immune response. The emotion immediately enters the meridian network as a powerful surge of intense energy-in-motion, charging wildly through the human energy system like a bull in a china shop, upsetting the internal organ-energies, draining glands, and disrupting the functional harmony of the whole system. By now beyond control by either body or mind, the emotion has become a rebellious aberrant energy that storms through the system and damages the internal terrain.

The Seven Emotions that cause "dis-ease" are joy, anger, anxiety, worry, grief, fear, and fright. Each is associated with a specific internal organ-energy and is governed by one of the Five Elemental Energies of nature, with corresponding relations to other energy factors. For convenience, these seven are sometimes reduced to five, with fear and fright (acute fear) listed together under Water and the kidney system, and anxiety and grief (acute anxiety) combined under Metal and the lung system.

All emotions trigger specific physiological responses throughout the entire human system by virtue of biofeedback between the endocrine and nervous systems, causing changes in pulse and blood pressure, stimulating or inhibiting respiration, and helping or hindering digestion, metabolism, immunity, and other vital functions. Normal, well-balanced emotional response runs its course through the energy system without doing any harm, while the highest, most spiritually edifying human emotions such as love, compassion, and devotion actually have positive healing effects in the body. We all know how wonderful we feel when we are in love, or devoted to a great master, or engaged in compassionate activites. Love and compassion generate very soothing, blissful energy that has the power to heal one's own body as well as others. Western scientists such as Marcel Vogel have recently been studying the remarkable healing powers of the particular internal energy frequencies produced in the human system by love, which indeed seems to have the power to conquer all.

But when negative emotions such as anger and grief prevail, and when emotional response is allowed to become extreme or explosive, it sets off a series of physiological reactions that does great harm to the vital organs and glands, inhibits vital functions, impairs immunity, lowers resistance, and flings open the gates to disease and degeneration. Frequent and prolonged bouts of anger, for example, disrupt and inflame liver energy, which eventually gives rise to liver disease, which in turn further predisposes the individual to more bouts of anger, in a vicious cycle of self-destruction. Similarly, prolonged grief harms the lungs and causes shallow, erratic breathing patterns, which in turn disrupt the pulse, inhibit circulation, impair metabolism, and suppress the immune response, rendering the system vulnerable to disease and degeneration. In Western medical terms, the self-destructive nature of negative or extreme emotional response might be called psychoneuropathology, which represents the reverse effect of the recently discovered "mind-over-matter" healing response known as psychoneuroimmunology (PNI).

Like the Six Evils, the Seven Emotions have even more dangerous modern manifestations produced by the pace and pressure of contemporary urban lifestyles. By far the most harmful of these new forms of negative emotional response is stress, a repressed fight-or-flight response that combines elements of anger, fear, grief, and worry. Through biofeedback, stress sweeps through the whole system and impairs virtually every vital function in the body, particularly the immune response. Chronic stress therefore gives rise to chronic immune deficiency, and this is the root cause of many chronic degenerative conditions today. Recall that modern artificial forms of the Six Evils, such as microwaves, electric power fields, televisions, office equipment, and household appliances, have also been shown to particularly inhibit immune response, then add the immunosuppressant effects of stress, and it is no wonder that immune deficiency is so easily acquired from modern industrialized lifestyles.

While aberrant external and internal energies account for most types of human disease and degeneration in traditional Chinese medicine, Chinese physicians also recognize a third category of miscellaneous causes known as "neither external nor internal" (*bu wai, bu nei*). This category includes unexpected causes such as accidents and traumatic wounds, insect and animal bites, parasites and poisons, as well as negligent lifestyle factors such as gluttony, poor nutrition, alcohol and drug abuse, wrong combinations of food and drink, sexual exhaustion, and insufficient exercise. In traditional China, this category of factors was responsible for relatively few ailments, because social and environmental conditions, diet and nutrition, sexual activity, and other basic lifestyle factors were not nearly as hazardous to human health as they are today. In today's world, with all its pollution and social disorder, denatured diets and chemical additives, stress and hyperactivity, lifestyle has become a major contributing factor in all causes of disease, degeneration, and premature death, rather than a preventive bulwark against them.

The human energy system is a highly sensitive, finely tuned instrument that responds like a weather vane to the subtlest shifts in the prevailing winds of the internal and external environments, reacting instantly to any changes in the ambient energies that influence the system. Any abnormal fluctuations in the external or internal energies associated with the human system always have disturbing repercussions on both the body and the mind, and if left uncorrected, they soon manifest as symptoms of disease. The normal biorhythmic fluctuations of nature cause normal biorhythmic responses in the human system, which adapts to the new energy patterns without harm to the body or mind. However, any sudden or extreme shifts in energy—such as aberrant or unseasonal weather, a blast of microwave radiation, a temper tantrum or wave of paranoia—provoke abnormal, distressing responses that distort human energy patterns and disrupt the whole system, creating the conditions of internal imbalance and disorder that always set the stage for the onset of disease.

Energy is the medium through which the conditions that predispose the system to disease and degeneration are established in the human body, and energy is also the vehicle through which traditional Chinese medicine works to cure disease, halt degeneration, and heal the body. If we bear in mind that all matter, including every cell and tissue in the body, is ultimately nothing more than condensed, highly organized energy, then it is easy to see that physical ailments are really nothing more than pathological reactions to the abnormal energy patterns caused by aberrant "weather" in the system. When fair weather and harmonious winds prevail in the human energy system, physical health flourishes and the mind is at ease. When storms, droughts, floods, and ill winds sweep through the internal terrain of body and mind, the garden of health inevitably suffers damage and "dis-ease." The only way to restore health and recover peace of mind is to create the conditions of internal balance that the energy system requires to heal itself and to synchronize the whole human system with the rhythms of nature and the cosmos, bringing the Three Powers of Heaven, Earth, and Humanity back into harmony.

4

Traditional Chinese Diagnosis

ONE OF THE MOST TELLING differences between modern Western and traditional Chinese medicine lies in their approaches to the diagnosis of disease. Western medicine focuses attention on the separate symptoms of disease, employing specialists and complex laboratory technology to pinpoint the precise location and analyze the exact pathology of each symptom, and to identify the particular microbes present in the affected area. This approach treats symptoms as though they were spontaneous, localized phenomena that occur independently from the rest of the body and it often fails to account for the hidden connections between overt symptoms in one part of the body and covert causes elsewhere, linked by the invisible webs of the human energy system. Western diagnosis often suggests the same treatment for the same symptom in all patients, overlooking critical constitutional variations among different patients' systems, and consequently, in Western therapeutics, one patient's medicine can be another's poison.

Traditional Chinese diagnosis views the external symptoms of disease as physiological reflections of internal imbalances in the energy system, and it uses them as indicators to track down the root causes of disease within the circuits of the human energy system. Chinese physicians utilize their own senses as diagnostic instruments, and they interpret their observations intuitively, based on clinical experience. First they diagnose the current status of the patient's whole system, looking for patterns of disharmony that might account for the pathology of the patient's various physical and mental symptoms, then they map out a strategy that corrects the conditions of imbalance responsible for the symptoms. Rather than simply suppressing separate symptoms with different drugs, as in Western allopathic medicine, Chinese medicine aims its therapies at correcting the systemic imbalance and functional disharmony that consititute the root cause of the whole condition, effecting a lasting cure and eliminating all abnormal symptoms in one therapeutic stroke.

Focusing primary attention on the unique patterns and prevailing conditions of each individual patient's whole system, rather than on the pathology and precise anatomical location of separate symptoms, is one of the most important diagnostic principles in traditional Chinese medicine, which views individual constitutional differences among patients suffering from the same ailments as being far more decisive factors in the diagnosis and treatment of disease than any superficial similarities among the symptoms they may experience in common. Everyone's internal organs may well look exactly alike in an autopsy or on the surgeon's table, but the way their vital energies and internal organs respond to external influences varies greatly from person to person, and these differences are decisive factors in the way a disease develops in a particular patient and how he or she will respond to a particular medical treatment. Chinese medicine recognizes that the same symptoms in different patients can have very different causes, and it accounts for these individual differences by prescribing "different strokes for different folks" in the application of medical therapies, rather than always using the same medicine for the same symptom in every patient, as allopathic Western doctors often do. This point is well made in the following passage from a Chinese medical treatise written in 1757, translated by Paul

Unschuld for a lecture he gave to the International Acupuncture Symposium in 1987:

> Illnesses may be identical but the persons suffering from them are different. . . . Some people may be strong and others weak as far as their energy or the condition of their body is concerned. . . . If one treats all those patients who appear to suffer from one identical illness with one and the same therapy, one may hit the nature of the illness but one's approach may still be exactly contraindicated by the influences of energy that determine the condition of the individual patient's body. . . . Physicians therefore must carefully take into account the differences among the people and only then decide whether the therapeutic pattern they employ suits . . . the individual constitution.

Chinese diagnosis has two stages. The first is the initial diagnosis of the current state of the patient's whole system, which serves as a framework for diagnosing the basic nature and root causes of the patient's particular symptoms. The second stage is called differential diagnosis, and this takes place during each subsequent visit to the doctor, to chart symptomatic changes during the course of treatment and track the progress of both the disease and the cure. This enables the physician to progressively adjust the therapies along the way, as the patient's symptoms shift and transform, and the system gradually regains its balance.

Both the initial and the subsequent differential stages of diagnosis employ two basic parameters to determine the cause and prescribe the cure for disease; these are known as the Four Diagnostics and the Eight Indicators. During the patient's first visit, the physician applies the Four Diagnostics to establish a complete picture of the current state of the patient's whole system, review his or her medical history, and analyze all symptoms within the overall context of the individual's inherent constitutional energy patterns. The Four Diagnostics are Questioning, Observing, Listening and Smelling, and Touching.

Questioning. The doctor requests a complete and detailed account of the patient's past and recent health history, asking probing questions about diet, exercise, hygiene, sleep, bowel movements, sexual activities, emotions, and other personal habits, then listening to the patient's specific complaints in light of his or her replies to all these questions.

Observing. The doctor scans the patient's body visually, looking for any abnormal signs in the patient's complexion, eyes, hair, nails, skin tone, and especially the color and condition of the tongue and tongue fur. The Chinese have refined tongue diagnosis to a fine art, recognizing twenty-four different conditions of internal energy imbalance based on the color and texture of tongue fur. Chinese diagnosis also reads the condition of five major organ-energy systems according to their corresponding zones on the tongue (fig. 6). The way the patient walks, sits,

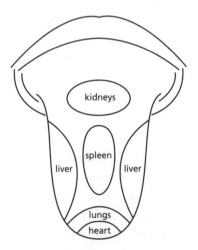

Figure 6. The zones of the tongue that reflect the conditions of the five yin organ-energy systems.

moves, gestures, breathes, twitches, and other subtle signs that
reflect internal energy conditions are all noted. The term *chee-
seh*, literally the "color of energy," refers to the overall condition of a patient's energy system, as observed by the physician,
as in "His energy color looks weak and pale," or "Her energy
color is bright and strong." It requires many years of clinical
experience to develop an accurate eye for the signs that indicate the "color" of a patient's energy.

Listening and smelling. These two appear together because in Chinese the same ideogram is used to denote the verbs *to smell*
and *to listen*, and Chinese physicians use both senses to take
measure of the patient's breath, timbre of voice, strength and
rhythm of pulse, intestinal rumblings, the smell of bodily secretions and excretions, and other signs of sound or smell by which
to gauge how energies and vital functions are working inside
the body.

Touching. This includes tactile examination of the patient's skin
and flesh, palpation of the internal organs and other tissues,
and pressing certain "alarm points" along the patient's meridian network to reveal disorders within the system. It also includes the most profoundly accurate, subtle, and uniquely
Chinese method of diagnosis—pressing pulses (*ba mai*)—
whereby the physician applies subtle pressures to three points
along the radial arteries of both wrists, detecting twelve different pulses that reflect the precise condition of each of the
twelve major organ-energy systems. It takes a very delicate
touch and long years of experience to master this ancient
method of pulse diagnosis, which can distinguish dozens of different energy patterns in each pulse, such as slippery, rapid,
empty, full, tight, wiry, knotted, skipping, shallow, and so forth.
But once the method is mastered, pulse diagnosis draws a complete and remarkably accurate picture of the patient's entire

internal system by revealing the precise conditions of each constituent organ system.

Through the Four Diagnostics, Chinese physicians use their own bodies as instruments to measure the patient's various vital signs, and they refer to their own clinical experience rather than manuals and laboratory tests to diagnose the data recorded by their senses and to prescribe an appropriate therapy. After therapy commences, the physician continues to monitor the course of the disease and track the progress of the cure with differential diagnosis, which follows symptoms as they move through the system during progressive stages of treatment. Differential diagnosis is based on various external signs of internal energy conditions known as the Eight Indicators; these indicators are yin and yang, internal and external, cold and hot, and empty and full.

Differential diagnosis is another unique hallmark of traditional Chinese medicine. It allows the physician periodically to adjust medical therapies to fit the ever-changing energy patterns within the patient's system as disease progresses through different stages of the cure. "Chinese medicine identifies disease as disorders of relationship, not as a singular, unvarying entity," write Beinfield and Korngold. "Problems recognized early on can be dealt with before they develop into complex, deep seated, chronic illness." By using yin and yang, the Five Elemental Energies, and the Eight Indicators to keep track of shifting symptoms as he or she rebalances the patient's whole system, the physician is able to apply precisely the right medicine to exactly the right organ-energy system at just the right time, working in close alliance with the body's own internal energies to chase the disorder out of the system. In this scenario, the doctor simply maps out the strategy and provides the patient with timely tactical aid, but it is up to the patient's own energies to fight the actual battle.

The Yellow Emperor's Classic of Internal Medicine states, "The good physician first diagnoses the condition in terms of yin and yang." Yin and yang are known in Chinese diagnosis as the Commanders of the Eight Indicators, because all the other indicators are simply different manifestations of yin and yang. External, hot, and full symptoms all indicate a basically yang condition, whereas internal, cold, and empty are signs of yin conditions. There are also many degrees and combinations in between the extremes of yin and yang. A cold symptom that manifests externally is called external-cold or yin within yang. A full symptom appearing internally is internal-full or yang within yin, and a hot symptom on the surface is external-hot or yang within yang, and so forth. Each combination of indicators calls for a particular therapeutic tactic. As *The Yellow Emperor's Classic* states, "If it's hot, cool it down; if it's cold, warm it up; if it's empty, fill it; if it's full, empty it." As the treatment progresses, the disease transforms through various stages and gives rise to different sets of symptomatic indicators that call for different therapeutics, until finally all indicators are balanced, all signs are normal, and a complete cure has been effected.

The Eight Indicators reflect the following basic symptomatic conditions:

Cold: depressed metabolic activity; aversion to cold; low body temperature; loose bowels; profuse light urine; lassitude and indifference

Hot: overactive metabolism; aversion to heat; high body temperature; constipation; scant, dark urine; nervous excitability and emotional instability

Empty: low resistance; impaired immune response; physical weakness; hypofunction of organ-energy systems; nervous exhaustion

Full: hyperfunction of organ-energy systems; hypersensitivity to stress and infection; high blood pressure; bloating

Internal: influencing internal organs and glands and deep tissues;

affecting the inside of body cavities; indicates serious internal stages in development of symptoms

External: influencing skin, hair, peripheral nerves, muscles, and tendons; affecting external surfaces and orifices; indicates superficial symptoms in the early stages of invasion or the final stages of elimination

Yin: composite conditions of cold, empty, and internal

Yang: composite conditions of hot, full, and external

Let us look at a few simple examples of how the Four Diagnostics and Eight indicators are used to diagnose the symptoms of disease in terms of yin and yang and the Five Elemental Energies, and how they are used to trace root causes to functional disorders and deficiencies in various vital organ-energy systems.

Say, for example, that an otherwise healthy man in his mid-forties comes to see a Chinese doctor about the high blood pressure and heart palpitations he has recently experienced for the first time in his life. Observation of external signs reveal no heart problems; the patient eats well and gets plenty of rest and exercise, and he is not subject to stress at home or work. Pulse diagnosis, however, indicates internal-empty yin conditions in the kidney system, which is governed by the elemental energy of Water, and under questioning during the interview the patient admits that he has recently indulged in a prolonged bout of wild sexual promiscuity, causing him to emit his semen almost every day. The doctor explains, "The excessive loss of semen and vital energy due to your recent activities has weakened your kidneys, which govern sexual energy, giving rise to an empty state of depletion in kidney-energy. According to the control cycle of the Five Elemental Energies, Water controls Fire. Since the Water energy in your kidneys has grown weak, it has lost control over the Fire energy in your heart, which has consequently flared out of control with full yang symptoms of high blood pressure and heart palpitations." Rather than prescribing drugs that provide quick but temporary relief by suppressing the symptoms of high blood pressure, as a Western physician might do, the Chinese doctor would get to the heart of the matter by prescribing herbs to tonify (i.e., "fill") the patient's empty kidney energy, while also recommending that the patient restrain his sexual activities to avoid emptying it again. When the patient's kidney energy has been fully restored, Water once again exerts its normal control over Fire, the heart calms down and recovers its natural rhythm, and all abnormal symptoms disappear.

Beinfield and Korngold give the following illustration of how the same basic symptom of headache can be diagnosed in very different ways in different patients, and traced to very different causes, depending on the "prevailing winds" in the individual patient's energy system:

> For example, disturbance of the *Liver Network* can produce migraine or bilious headaches associated with nausea, vomitting, and sensitivity to light and noise. These headaches may be provoked by anger and occur more frequently in the spring. Disturbance of the *Stomach* and *Intestines* may cause headaches associated with nasal and sinus congestion, acidity, flatulence, and constipation. This type of headache may appear in the morning and improve in the evening. Especially in hot, humid weather, disturbances of the *Spleen* and *Heart* may cause headaches associated with fatigue, dizziness, perspiration, and anxiety. In winter, headaches associated with backache, chilliness, and profuse urination may suggest a disturbance of the *Kidney*. The headache could be a simple matter of acute indigestion or related to a complex and chronic problem such as hypertension, asthma, allergies, or premenstrual syndrome. Treatment for someone's headache will differ according to which *Organ Network* is disturbed.

Chinese diagnosis is a selective analytical process that determines exactly what is happening when something goes wrong in the human energy system, how it relates to the various internal and external energies that influence the balance and harmony of the system, and why it is causing the particular symptoms in question. It employs all the principles and parameters of Chinese medicine—from yin and yang, the Three Treasures, and the Five Elemental Energies to the Six Evils, Seven Emotions, and Eight Indicators—to identify the underlying imbalance that is causing the ailment and to diagnose all symptoms within the context of the unique energy patterns prevailing in each individual patient's system. It is a dynamic process of spontaneous discovery that reveals exactly the right combination of therapeutic tactics to apply in each individual case, rather than always suggesting the same treatments for similar symptoms in all patients. By evaluating specific symptoms in light of the patient's whole system, Chinese diagnosis leaves no stone unturned in tracking down the root causes of disease, and all therapies are geared to enlist the patient's own internal energies to combat the condition and correct the imbalance. Treatment continues and therapies are periodically adjusted until all the abnormal conditions of energy imbalance that cause symptoms of disease are eliminated and functional harmony is restored to the whole system. If the course of treatment is properly followed and completed, a traditional Chinese cure will usually last for as long as the patient avoids the same mistakes and malevolent influences that caused the problem in the first place.

5

The Chinese Tree of Health

THE TRADITIONAL CHINESE SYSTEM of human health care is like a venerable old tree that has been growing continuously for thousands of years, its ancient roots firmly planted in the fertile soil of classical Taoist philosophy, its therapeutic branches spreading their soothing shade over the parched fields of human disease and degeneration. For all their colorful variety and different approaches to healing human maladies, every branch of the Chinese healing arts remains connected to the same main trunk of medical philosophy, and the same nourishing sap runs freely throughout the entire system of human health care. That sap is *chee*—the energy of life—in all its myriad manifestations, from the macrocosmic forces of nature and the cosmos down to the microcosmic energies that run like electric currents throughout all the organs, tissues, and cells of the human body. Energy remains the common denominator in all the complex equations of human health and disease, and each branch of the traditional Chinese healing arts deals with the fundamental energies of Heaven, Earth, and Humanity (the Three Powers) with a holistic approach that restores their primordial harmony.

Unlike modern Western medicine, which has grown increasingly fragmented into narrowly specialized departments focused exclusively on specific parts of the body or particular categories of disease, traditional Chinese medicine offers the patient a variety of different ways to heal and rebalance the whole system in order to cure all types of ailments. All these various methods, such as herbs and nutrition, acupuncture and massage, exercise and meditation, are wholly synergistic and may be applied in harmonious conjunction with one another. By contrast, the specialists of modern Western medicine are trained to deal with only one part of the human system or one type of disease, with very little cross-reference and virtually no common ground in practical therapeutics. In traditional Chinese medical practice, the same physician is called on to handle gynecological problems, prostate conditions, childhood respiratory disorders, and the neurological dysfunctions of the old and senile. In modern Western medicine, a woman must seek the services of a gynecologist, a man with prostate problems must go to a urologist, children are sent to pediatricians, and the elderly go to gerontological neurologists.

The major difference between the traditional Eastern and modern Western approaches to health is that the traditional Eastern way deals with any and all symptoms within the organic context of the whole human system, seeking and treating root causes wherever they may lie hidden within the system in order to achieve a lasting cure, while the Western method seems to focus too often only on the part of the body where overt symptoms appear, providing swift but only temporary relief from symptomatic discomforts while overlooking hidden causes elsewhere in the body. Traditional Chinese physicians must therefore become qualified to practice all branches of the tree of Chinese therapy, and they must understand all aspects of the whole human system, while Western specialists are trained mainly to deal with isolated parts or specific conditions. The result of this difference is that Chinese therapies generally take longer to work but usually provide lasting cures, while Western therapies provide quick relief at the cost of future relapses. The latter way involves an ever-escalating cycle of complications that lead to lifelong dependence on doctors and drugs and often end up requiring radical surgical excision of damaged parts.

The difference between the organic, holistic approach of traditional Chinese therapy and the specialized, fragmented method of modern Western treatments is clearly reflected in the preparation and training required to become a qualified practitioner. Whereas most Western medical doctors require only four to five years of formal training to become licensed in their chosen specialty, it takes an average of ten to twelve years of rigorous study and clinical apprenticeship to become fully qualified to practice traditional Chinese medicine in China, Taiwan, Hong Kong, and other East Asian countries. Chinese physicians must become familiar with all branches of the Chinese tree of health, and, in many cases, they must be able to apply two or more types of therapy to treat their patients' conditions. Patients benefit greatly from this holistic approach because they can take all their health problems to one doctor and follow a systematic, organic healing program that corrects all their disorders at the same time. This systematic approach saves patients a lot of time, trouble, and expense; more often than not, if the patient faithfully complies with the prescribed regimen, it eventually affects a complete and lasting cure.

The tree of traditional Chinese health care is therefore an integrated system of synergistic therapies in which each branch stems from the same root principles and utilizes the same basic energies on which all forms of life depend. Although each branch employs different therapeutic tools to deal with various health problems and constitutional deficiencies, they all work in concert toward achieving the ultimate goal of restoring optimum energy balance and functional harmony to the whole system, as well as establishing equilibrium between the whole human system and the environmental elements and energies that shape and nurture it. "Chinese medical thinking integrates medicine, whose aim is to heal the body and mind, with philosophy, whose purpose is to guide us in living," write

Beinfield and Korngold. "The insights of Chinese medicine can nurse our sense of ourselves, our awareness, at the same time as acupuncture and herbs can promote our direct experience of integration." It is this sense of integration between body and mind, internal and external energies, macrocosmic and microcosmic forces, experienced through a harmonious balance among all the energies of life, that constitutes traditional Chinese medicine's greatest gift to human health and happiness.

6
Herbal Medicine

HERBAL MEDICINE IS BY FAR the oldest and most richly foliated branch on the Chinese tree of health and healing. References to medicinal herbs appear frequently in the earliest annals of Chinese history, including the ancient *Book of Change* (*I-Ching*) and the *Book of Odes* (*Shih Ching*), two of the sacred early Chou dynasty classics annotated by Confucius. In the latter, we find poetic descriptions of young maidens singing in the hills and valleys as they gather medicinal herbs for pharmaceutical use at home. So prevalent was the daily use of medicinal herbs in the households of ancient China that to this day one of the most common ways of saying "What's wrong with you?" in Chinese is, "Did you eat the wrong medicine today?"

In the strict Western definition, the word *herb* refers only to plants and plant-derived extracts, but in Chinese medicine it also includes minerals and animal products—that is, anything derived from nature's cornucopia. The use of medicinal minerals has a long and colorful history in China, and Chinese physicians were early to recognize the vital role that minerals play in human metabolism, particularly as conductors and catalysts for the electromagnetic currents of the human energy system. Often employed as sedatives in the Calm Spirit (*ding shen*) category of herbal medicine, medicinal minerals find frequent use in a wide range of nervous disorders. They also constitute the main active ingredients in many of the famous longevity elixirs (*chang shou dan*) concocted by Taoist alchemists and wizards for their imperial patrons, some of whom lost their lives prematurely while trying to prolong them with toxic mineral prescriptions. Medicinal minerals are similarly employed in the renowned "long-life pills" prepared in Ayurvedic and traditional Tibetan medicine.

Perhaps the most important mineral substance traditionally used in longevity and nervous-system formulas is cinnabar (*ju sha*), a highly refined extract of mercury that is still prescribed in formulas for hypertension, insomnia, anxiety, shock, and other nervous disorders. In minute doses, cinnabar acts as a powerful sedative, antispasmodic, and nerve tonic, but in higher doses or with prolonged use it can become quite toxic to the human system. Other mineral substances commonly employed for their sedative effects include oyster shell (*mu li*), magnetite (*tse shih*), and fossilized dinosaur bones (*lung gu*). Sea salt (*hai yen*) is also an excellent source of medicinal minerals, particularly magnesium and trace elements. Due to the presence of balancing trace elements, sea salt does not cause the hypertension and renal problems associated with the refined, mined table salt sold in modern markets, even when used for daily culinary purposes.*

Animal products are another class of Chinese herbal medicine rarely encountered in the Western medical tradition. Centipedes and scorpions, earthworms and snakes, praying mantises and silkworms, tortoise shell and deer horn—all play major roles in many traditional Chinese herbal formulas, and their medical efficacy ranks them among the most highly prized substances in the Chinese pharmacopeia, particularly in the tonic category.

---

*See Jacques de Langre, *Seasalt's Hidden Powers* (Magalia, Calif.: Happiness Press, 1994).

Tonics are a special category of Chinese herbal medicine that are meant primarily for preventive use by healthy individuals, not for curative purposes by the sick. Virtually all tonic herbs fall into the Superior (*shang*) class of medicinal herbs, which means that they have proven efficacy as protectors of health and promoters of longevity in humans, without any toxic side effects. These life-prolonging properties have made tonics the favorite herbs of emperors and generals, ministers and magistrates, and this demand has rendered them among the most expensive items in the Chinese pharmacopeia. Tonics were also well known in traditional Western medicine until the turn of the twentieth century, when chemical drugs and surgery eradicated their use as preventive medicine in health care.

Tonic animal products—such as deer horn and sea horse, tortoise shell and donkey hide—contain potent proteins and hormone residues that have strong stimulating effects on the human endocrine system, promoting glandular secretions that energize the whole system and activate flagging vital functions, particularly sexual vitality, immune response, and cerebral functions. Such well-known plant-derived tonics are ginseng, astragalus, and codonopsis are what Western herbology refers to as "adaptogens," which means that they naturally adapt the vital functions of the human system to compensate for adverse conditions such as stress, malnutrition, aberrant environmental energies, and the degenerative conditions associated with aging, thereby preventing somatic damage and prolonging the life of the whole organism. Adaptogenic tonics work primarily by tonifying blood factors, stimulating vital organ-energies, and balancing yin and yang throughout the whole system.

Another category of herbal remedy that is unique to Chinese medicine comprises the constitutional formulas, which have both preventive and curative properties. These formulas are specifically designed to correct particular problems caused by individual constitutional deficiencies and energy imbalances that are inherited prenatally or acquired postnatally through personal lifestyles and habits.

Virtually everyone on earth has a certain degree of inherent imbalance or distortion among their vital energies and organic functions, and these constitutional disparities account for many minor aches and pains and chronic conditions that most Westerners either take for granted or try in vain to cure with allopathic drugs. However, it does little good—and often does long-term harm—to take drugs for symptomatic relief of chronic discomforts whose root causes lie in deep-seated constitutional deficiencies. On the other hand, constitutional herbal formulas that are custom-prepared to compensate for such deficiencies can rebalance one's entire organ-energy network, not only relieving the associated symptomatic discomforts, but also correcting the underlying constitutional causes. Here are a few common examples of how such formulas work.

- Chronic mental fatigue, frequent headaches, insomnia, and absentmindedness are often symptomatic signs of an inherent or acquired constitutional deficiency in cerebral circulation. Rather than taking aspirin, amphetamines, sleeping pills, and other drugs for such problems, one could alleviate the entire syndrome with a single constitutional formula that enhances cerebral circulation, using such herbs as gotu kola, ginkgo, ginseng, and schisandra.
- A middle-aged man who has led an excessively promiscuous life in his youth and now suffers from chronic lumbago, frequent urination, painful, weak knees, and cold extremities has acquired a constitutional deficiency of kidney-yin and would generally benefit from taking the famous patent kidney-yin formula called Six Flavor Rehmannia Pills (*liu wei di huang wan*).
- A woman with chronic menstrual problems such as dysmenorrhea and PMS due to an inherent constitutional blood deficiency would find both symptomatic relief and a possible long-term cure by taking a custom-formulated prescription based on the great female blood tonic *Angelica sinensis* (*dang gui*).

All Chinese herbs act therapeutically on the targeted organs and tissues by virtue of their natural affinity (*gui jing*, literally "home into meridians") for the energy channels that govern those organs and tissues. The therapeutic activity of Chinese herbs thus functions more on the level of energy than chemistry, although they also have direct biochemical effects. The unique frequency and valence of molecular energy within each herbal essence determines its particular organ affinity by resonating in synchronicity with the frequency and valence of the molecules within the tissues of the particular organ targeted for treatment. Through thousands of years of continuous clinical observation, Chinese medical science has identified the specific organ-energy affinities of thousands of medicinal herbs and foods. Similar observations have been recorded in the herbal medical traditions of India, Persia, medieval Europe, and native North and South American tribes, all of which basically agree on the therapeutic properties of medicinal herbs they share in common. By combining various herbs in compound formulas, a remarkable degree of specificity and combined effects can be achieved to deal with the particular problems of individual patients. This method is far superior to the modern allopathic practice of simply prescribing the same chemical drug for the same basic condition in all patients.

Chinese medical herbs are classified according to their basic yin-yang nature (warming, cooling, or neutral), their Five Elemental Energy identities as reflected in the Five Flavors (pungent, sweet, sour, bitter, or salty), and their primary therapeutic properties (tonifying, purging, concentrating, or dispersing) (table 4). These various classifications combine to determine the precise therapeutic functions and pharmacodynamic effects of each individual herb in the Chinese pharmacopeia, based on thousands of years of continuous empirical observation and clinical application, and they are matched in therapeutic practice against the symptomatic signs and constitutional requirements of each individual patient's system. Whenever a new herb comes to the attention of Chinese herbalists, such as from

TABLE 4. The Five Flavors and Related Attributes of Chinese Medicinal Herbs

Flavor	Elemental energy	Organ affinity	Theraputic effects	Example
Pungent	Metal	Lungs/large intestine	Stimulating, diaphoretic, dispersing, clears stagnation	Ginger, clove, garlic
Sweet	Earth	Spleen/ stomach	Nourishing, digestive, harmonizing	Licorice, honey, Job's tears
Sour	Wood	Liver/ gallbladder	Astringent, concentrating, antipyretic	Rhubarb, plum, peony
Bitter	Fire	Heart/small intestine	Drying, purging, antidote, cooling	Loquat, lotus leaf, gentian
Salty	Water	Kidney/ bladder	Softening, diuretic, laxative, dissolving	Seaweed, mirabilite, deer horn

Europe or the Americas, it is immediately identified in terms of its fundamental Five Elemental Energy category, based on the obvious attribute of flavor, but its other pharmaceutical properties take many years of clinical practice to establish.

Traditional Chinese herbalists have developed a number of different methods of preparing both single herbs and compound formulas for internal and external application. The method of preparation used for each remedy depends on several factors, including the nature of the herb(s), the type of condition to be treated, and the therapeutic effects to be achieved. Below is a brief description of the most commonly employed modes of preparing Chinese herbs for therapeutic use.

Raw

Eating herbs in the fresh, raw state is the original and most ancient method of ingesting herbs for medicinal purposes. The emperor Shen Nung ("Divine Farmer"), legendary founder of Chinese herbal medicine, is often depicted chomping on a handful of fresh raw herbs, and it is said he thus tasted and tested seventy herbs per day until he had established the pharmacological properties of all the medicinal herbs in the Chinese empire. Many medicinal herbs are most potent when taken raw, but others require drying, cooking, soaking, washing with vinegar, and other types of processing to neutralize toxic constituents or activate pharmacological properties, so it is not a good idea to experiment on your own with freshly gathered raw herbs without the guidance of a qualified herbalist. Unless you have such guidance, or formal training in Chinese herbology, you should always purchase your medicinal herbs from a reputable Chinese pharmacy or herbal supplier and use them according to professional instructions.

Decoction

The most traditional and popular method of preparing medicinal herbs for use at home is to boil a decoction (*tang*, literally "broth") of dried herbs in an earthenware or heat-proof glass vessel, simmering the brew until the liquid is reduced by about half. This method ensures maximum extraction of the herbs' full medicinal properties, rapid assimilation, and quick therapeutic effects, which makes this the best method for most acute conditions. The only drawback is that it requires you to spend some time each day in the kitchen.

An adaptation of this method is steam decoction, whereby a lidded ceramic bowl containing the herb(s) and a few ounces of pure water is set on a rack inside a larger vessel, and the herbs are steamed for several hours. Also known as a ginseng cooker, this method yields a very pure, potent extract called medicinal dew (*yao lu*) and is most suitable for expensive tonic herbs such as old ginseng, prepared either singly or in simple combination, but not for complex bulk formulas.

Powder

Powders (*san*) can be prepared at home from dried herbs with an electric coffee grinder, or at the pharmacy, but either way they should be freshly ground in sufficient quantities for no more than two or three weeks, so they do not lose their potency. Powders act more slowly and gently than decoctions or fresh raw herbs, and their effects last longer, which makes them most suitable for chronic conditions requiring long-term therapy.

There are three ways to take powders. The simplest and most traditional way is to spoon the required dose into your mouth and wash it down with warm water or warm wine, such as Japanese sake or mild sherry. Another traditional method is to place the measured dose of powder in a cup and pour hot water over it to make an infusion (*cha*). The third and most modern way is to stuff the powdered herbs into gelatin capsules (*jiau niang*), which is highly convenient and particularly useful for taking bitter, hard-to-swallow powders.

Pastes

Pastes (*gao*) are prepared by blending powdered herbs with just enough honey to form an herbal dough, which is then eaten by the spoonful and chased down with warm water or wine. Pastes may be stored for many months in sealed jars in the refrigerator.

Pills

Pills (*wan*) are prepared from honey herbal paste by rolling small pellets between thumb and index finger, then placing them on a baking sheet and putting them in an oven at the lowest temperature for about fifteen minutes, until they begin to glaze. After they cool completely, they may be stored in tightly sealed brown jars for many months, without refrigeration. Typical doses are five to fifteen pills taken two or three times daily with warm water or wine. Unlike Western tablets, Chinese honey pills are made without excipients, fillers, preservatives, or other nonherbal additives. Some types of pills are made with other natural bases, such as water, beeswax, or fermented flour dough.

Liquors

Herbal liquor (*yao jiou*) is prepared by steeping whole or roughly chopped dried herbs in strong distilled spirits such as vodka for two to four months or up to a full year, depending on the formula. This is an ancient and very efficient way of extracting full medicinal potential from expensive tonic herbs such as ginseng, deer horn, seahorse, and other potent tonics. Also known as Spring Wine, tonic herbal liquors may be prepared at home or purchased ready-made in attractive decanters, and they are renowned for their rejuvenating effects and swift energizing properties.

Ointments

Herbal ointments (*yio*) are prepared for external use by blending finely powdered herbs in a warm oil base, such as sesame or almond oil, yellow Vaseline, lard, lanolin, or beeswax. They may be stored long-term in well-lidded jars without refrigeration. The most popular commercial herbal ointment is Tiger Balm.

Suppositories

Herbal suppositories (*sai ji*) are an ancient Chinese form of medication first referred to in Chang Chung-ching's *Discussion of Fevers and Flus*, written during the early Han dynasty. They are prepared by blending aromatic powdered herbs in a honey base to form small herbal bullets.

Extracts and Tinctures

Herbal extracts and tinctures (*yao jing*) are a more recent method of preparation using modern pharmaceutical extraction techniques. Very pure and highly concentrated, Chinese extracts and tinctures are always made from the whole plant, preferably fresh and raw, never from isolated fragments as in modern Western pharmacology. These full-spectrum extracts contain all sorts of natural synergists, many of them as yet unidentified, that balance the effects of the main active constituents and prevent the toxic reactions and other unpleasant side effects often experienced with fractional extracts and concentrates.

In Chinese herbal medicine, most compound formulas are combined according to a traditional system known as the Four Responsible Roles, in which each constituent herb plays a specific functional role in the therapeutic activities of the whole formula. The principal active herb in any formula is known as the King, and it is selected for its primary therapeutic action in the patient's condition. This is always the strongest herb in the formula, and in complex formulas for acute ailments, there are often two or three King herbs.

The secondary herb or herbs is called the Minister, and it has similar but complementary effects to the King, giving the formula a broader range of efficacy. The third role is called Assistant, and there are usually several of these herbs added to the formula to neutralize any toxic constituents in the primary herbs, counteract undesirable side effects of the whole formula, and enhance the major therapeutic actions of the King and Minister herbs.

The fourth role is known as the Servant, and its function is to harmonize the overall effects of the entire formula and facilitate rapid assimilation and thorough distribution throughout the system. Servant herbs also prolong the effects of the primary ingredients, and are sometimes added to provide swift relief of symptomatic discomforts while the King and Minister herbs work gradually to correct the root cause of the condition.

Today, the ancient art and science of Chinese herbal medicine continues its five-thousand-year-old tradition of research and development, based on ongoing clinical practice and empirical observation in China as well as in other countries where Chinese medicine is now practiced as alternative therapy, such as America, Australia, and Western Europe. With the analytical assistance of modern laboratory technology and improved methods of extraction and refinement, all sorts of new uses for old herbs and new versions of traditional formulas are being developed specifically to deal with the unique health problems of contemporary times—particularly cancer, AIDS, and many chronic degenerative disorders associated with industrial society.

Cinnamon, for example, which has been used in Chinese medicine for thousands of years as a warming yang tonic, has recently been shown to significantly boost the effectiveness of insulin in people with diabetes. Several scientific studies have demonstrated cinnamon to enhance the activity of insulin in living cells by nearly 1,200 percent! "That's very important," says biochemist Richard Anderson of the U.S. Department of Agriculture's Human Nutrition Research Center, "because most secondary problems diabetics get, like cardiovascular disease, are the result of elevated insulin use. We've already heard from diabetics saying that they've seen definite improvement by using half a teaspoon of cinnamon a day."

Another interesting remedy for contemporary problems is a formula for drug addiction developed in China at the People's Liberation Army No. 1 Medical College. Based on a mixture of more than 40 traditional Chinese herbs, the formula is reported to relieve the intense symptoms of drug withdrawal within thirty minutes of administration and to achieve clinical abstinence in three to five days of therapy. Doctors in China claim that the formula, which is effective for heroin, morphine, and opium addiction, as well as amphetamines and other pharmaceutical drugs, has shown a 95 percent success rate in preliminary studies over a period of five years, according to Chinese reports.

Similar herbal remedies are being researched and developed in China, Japan, and certain Western countries for various types of cancer, AIDS and related immune deficiency syndromes, Parkinson's disease and other central nervous system disorders, and many other contemporary conditions, and the positive results of this work have placed traditional herbal medicine on the cutting edge of modern medical research.

One of the most practical modern developments in Chinese herbal medicine is the growing variety and availability of patent herbal formulas for a wide range of common health disorders. Over-the-counter patent remedies first appeared in China during the Sung dynasty (960–1279 CE), and today there are hundreds of convenient and inexpensive formulas available throughout the world. Some, such as the famous Six Flavor Rehmannia Pills (*liu wei di huang wan*), are ancient tried-and-true formulas that have been in continuous use for many centuries, while others are modern variations of traditional formulas developed by talented Western herbalists such as Charlie Jordan of Dragon River Herbal in New Mexico. American herbalist Jake Fratkin has written a very useful guide to these patent remedies, entitled *Chinese Herbal Patent Formulas: A Practical Guide,* which includes both Chinese classics and contemporary American variations.

For those who have never tried any herbal remedies, Chinese patent formulas can have truly dramatic effects and turn even the staunchest skeptic into a confirmed believer by delivering swift results, effective relief, and lasting cures for many common ailments, without the unpleasant side effects often associated with modern chemical drugs. Uninitiated readers who wish to give these patent remedies a try might start with some of the following famous formulas:

Yin Chiao Pien (Honeysuckle and Forsythia Tablets): For colds and flu of the "hot" variety, with symptoms of sneezing, runny nose, sore, swollen throat, fever, headache, and stiff neck and shoulders, this formula can provide almost miraculous relief if taken at the very first onset of symptoms and continued for two to three days. It can often knock out in two to three days what might otherwise become a two-to-three-week bout of respiratory misery, without the unpleasant side effects of antihistamines, decongestants, and other so-called cold remedies touted by Western pharmaceutical companies.

Gan Mao Ling (Common Cold Remedy): Another excellent remedy for common colds that can nip a bad cold in the bud if taken at the first sign of symptoms, this one is most appropriate for curing the sort of cold associated with chills. It can also be used to help prevent colds when you think you might become exposed to them.

Kang Ning Wan (Curing Pills): This is an excellent remedy for all sorts of common digestive disorders, such as acid indigestion, gas, nausea, toxic food reactions (including MSG syndrome), overeating, hangovers, and stomach flu. It is a cheap, effective, and highly versatile remedy for all sorts of gastric malaise caused by bad food and drink, or improper eating habits.

Bao Ji Wan (Po Chai Pills): Another effective remedy for the digestive disorders listed above, it may also be used by children, the elderly, and those with weak or impaired digestive systems. Both this and Curing Pills are great digestive aids to take along when traveling, and can be used as preventive remedies when you think you might become exposed to contaminated food and water.

Liu Wei Di Huang Wan (Six Flavor Rehmannia Pills): One of the most popular classic formulas of all time, this patent is an excellent overall tonic remedy for exhausted kidney, spleen, and liver yin-energy, with symptoms such as chronic fatigue, lower-back pain, night sweats, insomnia, male impotence, frequent urination, tinnitus (ringing ears), and high blood pressure. It is particularly effective for middle-aged men who experience the above symptoms as a result of excessive loss of semen due to undisciplined sexual activities in their youth.

Yunnan Bai Yao (Yunnan White Powder): Prized as an herbal treasure for centuries by China's military men and martial artists, this powder will swiftly stanch even the most traumatic bleeding wounds and facilitate rapid healing of tissues with minimal scarring. Taken internally, it stops internal hemorrhaging and may be used effectively before and after surgery to minimize bleeding, bruising, and swelling, as well as for excessive menstrual bleeding, hemorrhoids, bleeding ulcers, sprains, and gum infections. This patent remedy was standard issue in the field kits of all North Vietnamese troops during the Vietnam War and enabled them to dress their own gunshot wounds in the field.

Chinese herbal medicine, which has been in continuous use for at least five thousand years, is a safe and effective alternative to the increasingly toxic chemical drugs currently promoted in modern medical practice by allopathic doctors and pharmaceutical companies. In 1992, for example, the Annual Report of the American Association of Poison Control Centers reported not one single death or injury from the use of medicinal herbs in the United States, while during the same year, ten million people reported adverse effects, many of them life-threatening, from the use of pharmaceutical drugs approved by the FDA and routinely prescribed by conventional American physicians. The repeated efforts by the FDA, the AMA, and other American medical authorities to restrict public access to herbs and nutritional supplements is therefore completely unjustified and irrational and can only be viewed as an attempt to protect vested pharmaceutical and allopathic medical interests by denying the public the right to freely purchase herbs that can be successfully and inexpensively used to treat many common disorders at home, without resort to doctors or drugs. One obvious reason for this interference is that neither herbs nor nutrients can be patented and monopolized for profit by private corporate interests, as all chemical drugs are.

As the World Health Organization states in its "Guidelines for the Assessment of Herbal Medicines" (1992), "A guiding principle should be that if the product has been traditionally used without demonstrated harm, no specific restrictive regulatory action should be undertaken unless new evidence demands a revised risk-benefit assessment." This principle clearly applies to the herbal branch of traditional Chinese medicine, which has provided manifold health benefits to billions of users for thousands of years without any demonstrated harm or long-term risks—a claim that certainly cannot be made for modern pharmaceutical drugs, radiation therapy, radical surgery, and other modern medical procedures so routinely applied to patients today.

7
Diet and Nutrition

IN TRADITIONAL CHINESE THERAPY there is no fixed boundary between food and medicine, and whenever possible, illness is cured first by nutrition. As the famous Tang dynasty physician Sun Ssu-miao wrote fourteen centuries ago in his great medical treatise *Precious Recipes*, "The truly good physician . . . first treats the patient with food; only when food fails does he resort to drugs."

Prior to the advent of modern allopathic medicine in the early decades of the twentieth century, nutritional therapy was also a guiding principle in Western medicine. Hippocrates, the father of Western medicine, echoed Sun Ssu-miao's words when he taught his students, "Thy food shall be thy medicine." The renowned American doctor Charles Mayo wrote, "Normal resistance to disease is directly dependent upon adequate food. Normal resistance to disease *never* comes out of pill boxes." The celebrated American naturopath Harvey Kellogg adamantly opposed the substitution of chemical drugs for proper nutrition that occurred so rapidly in Western medicine during the early twentieth century, and he successfully used diet and nutrition, proper food combining, fasting and colon cleansing, and other dietary methods to cure thousands of patients of all types of disease and degenerative conditions at his sanitarium in Battle Creek, Michigan.

Chinese medicine has recognized the therapeutic value of food for thousands of years, and today strict dietary discipline remains an important aspect of treatment in all branches of traditional Chinese therapy. Because of their inherent medicinal properties and active energies, foods can easily enhance or obstruct the therapeutic benefits of herbs, acupuncture, and other types of treatment, and therefore compliance with the dietary guidelines always given by Chinese physicians remains a crucial factor in the efficacy of all Chinese therapies.

Like everything else in traditional Chinese medicine, diet and nutrition boil down to the basic principles of yin and yang and the Five Elemental Energies. The pharmacodynamic properties of food are identified according to the Four Energies of yin and yang (cool and cold, warm and hot) and the Five Flavors aspect of the Five Elemental Energies (sweet/Earth, pungent/Metal, salty/Water, sour/Wood, and bitter/Fire). The yin-yang classification determines a food's overall influence on the human energy system, with warm and hot yang foods stimulating vital organs and glands and increasing internal heat, cool and cold yin foods calming and cooling the system. The Five Flavor classification identifies the food's natural affinity for various organs, with sweet/Earth foods such as corn and dates entering the spleen/stomach meridians, pungent/Metal foods like ginger and garlic influencing the lung/large intestine system, sour/Wood foods going to the liver and gallbladder, and so forth. Chinese physicians dispense dietary advice to achieve optimum balance within the patient's whole system and also to target specific organ-energy systems for therapeutic treatment.

Whereas modern Western medicine views food simply in terms of its biochemical constituents and suggests eating "a bit of everything at every meal" to achieve a so-called balanced diet, Chinese doctors look at food in terms of the types of energy it releases into the human system. They then try to balance those energies with the individual patient's particular medical requirements and constitutional nature. What might be one patient's medicine could easily be another's poison, and therefore it is dietary folly to simply advise all patients to eat the same basic foods at every meal. A person with a hot yang constitution would benefit from eating plenty of cooling yin foods such as raw vegetable salads, but someone with an excess of yin should avoid raw foods altogether and eat more stimulating yang foods, such as fish and grains.

Another important aspect of balancing the diet for optimum therapeutic value is the fine science of food combining, known as trophology in Western terminology, a science long forgotten in modern Western medical practice. Chinese medicine has understood the vital role of proper food combining in human health and longevity for a long time, and most Chinese still practice it when eating at home or in restaurants. In 1378, on the occasion of his own hundredth birthday, the Taoist adept Chia Ming presented the founding emperor of the Ming dynasty with a book entitled *Essential Knowledge for Eating and Drinking*. In it he wrote:

> Food and drink are relied upon to nurture life. But if one does not know that the natures of substances may be opposed to each other, and one consumes them altogether indiscriminately, the vital organs will be thrown out of harmony and disastrous consequences will soon arise. Those who wish to nurture their lives must carefully avoid doing such damage to themselves.

The most basic principle of proper food combining is to avoid conflicts of yin and yang in the stomach. In Western terms, this is known as alkaline and acid, or pH, balance. When foods that require an acid medium of digestive enzymes in the stomach—such as meat, eggs, and other concentrated proteins—are eaten together with foods that require an alkaline medium, such as bread, rice, noodles, and other carbohydrates, the two types of digestive enzymes conflict and neutralize each other, forming a neutral medium that digests neither type of food. Instead, the carbohydrates ferment and the proteins putrefy, causing gas, acid indigestion, flatulence, heartburn, and all sorts of other digestive distress. Even the Hebrew scriptures contain clear references to the wisdom of proper food combining. Among the laws Moses handed down to his people was one that stipulated that they "shall eat flesh" in the evening and "be filled with bread" in the morning—that is, they should consume their proteins and carbohydrates separately. These laws also forbade the consumption of meat and milk at the same meal, and this remains one of the most basic axioms in the science of food combining. While meat and milk are both forms of protein, they have entirely different digestive requirements in the stomach, and if consumed together they can cause serious digestive disorders due to putrefaction. Yet today, the "Standard American Diet" (SAD)—as modern American eating habits are known in the contemporary literature of alternative nutritional medicine in America—includes meat and potatoes, hamburgers and french fries, eggs and toast, and all sorts of other digestively disastrous combinations of food to be eaten together for breakfast, lunch, and dinner, all washed down with cow's milk and orange juice, and followed by sweet, sugary desserts that really gum up the digestive tract. Small wonder that over 50 percent of the American population suffers from some form of chronic digestive distress, and that obesity has become a national phenomenon.

Generally, animal products and most grains are acid-forming yang foods, whereas fruits and vegetables are alkaline-forming yin, but some types of yang foods have alkaline properties, and some yin foods, which usually tend to be alkaline, have acid-forming properties (fig. 7). The ideal dietary balance for the human system is 80 percent alkaline to 20 percent acid foods, and this is what the traditional Chinese diet generally achieved prior to the infusion of modern Western products such as dairy, junk, and fast foods. By contrast,

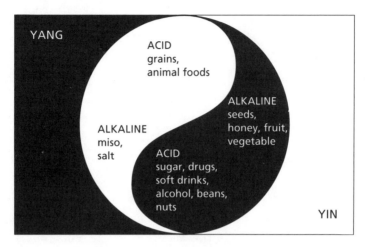

Figure 7. Yin and yang categories of food.

the SAD runs about 80 percent acid to 20 percent alkaline, resulting in a chronic state of acidification of the bloodstream and internal organs known as acidosis. Acidosis is responsible for many types of chronic degenerative disorders that Western physicians mistake for ailments rather than symptoms of improper dietary habits, including arthritis, tooth and bone degeneration, chronic fatigue, heart and circulatory problems, intestinal disorders, and many more.

One of the most therapeutically beneficial foods on nature's menu is mushrooms, which have played a prominent role in the Chinese diet for thousands of years. The medical properties of mushrooms have been well known in China since the dawn of civilization there. In recent years, research scientists in China and Japan have found potent anticarcinogenic properties in over fifty varieties of mushrooms, most notably the shitake, maitake, and reishi, which inhibit the formation of tumors and stimulate strong immune response throughout the human system. Other types of fungi, such as black and white Tree Ears, can be used to cure and prevent a wide range of chronic ailments, including arteriosclerosis, *Candida* infection, high blood pressure, and others.

Recently, a tea made from a fungus known as Kombucha has become a popular rejuvenative tonic in New Age health circles. This fungus originated in ancient China, from where it spread early to Korea. In 414 CE, a Korean physician named Kombu brought it to Japan, and ever since it has been known as Kombu-cha (*cha* means "tea" in Chinese as well as Japanese). Kombucha, which must be prepared at home from a starter fungus, is an excellent preventive tonic that benefits virtually every major organ-energy system in the body. It may also be used to purge the body of accumulated toxic residues, purify the bloodstream, and cure many common degenerative conditions.

In addition to their biochemical nutritional constituents, such as vitamins, minerals, and amino acids, fresh whole foods also contain the Five Elemental Energies of nature in condensed, crystalline forms, and these energies are released into the human energy system when digested and metabolized. Plants, for example, transform and store Fire energy from the sun, Water energy from water, Earth energy from soil, and Metal energy from minerals, and these energies are released to nourish the related organ-energy systems within the human body when the plant foods are consumed. Human health relies as much on these essential energies of nature as it does on biochemical nutrients, and indeed the two forms of nutrition are inseparably linked. Chlorophyll, for example, which transforms and stores the Fire energy of the sun in plants, differs in molecular structure by only one atom from hemoglobin, which carries oxygen in the human bloodstream. All fresh green foods therefore cleanse and tonify the blood, which is related in the Chinese medical paradigm to the Fire energy of the heart. Only fresh whole foods contain the vital energies of nature on which human health depends, and that is why modern diets denatured of all their living energies by factory processing and artificial additives fail to deliver the sort of essential energies that the human body requires to function properly.

In his book *Spiritual Tradition and the Rainbow Diet,* Dr. Gabriel Cousens explains the energetic properties of foods as follows:

> Within the plant structure, there are different crystallinelike substructures, similar to the multiple oscillating crystalline-like subsystems in our own bodies. These resonate with the bone and other crystallinelike structures in our bodies. . . . In this way, specific vibrational properties of the plant energize and nurture specific organ, glandular, and cellular systems.

This is a modern scientific way of describing how the Five Elemental Energies contained in fresh whole foods enter various associated organ-energy systems of the human body by virtue of their natural affinity for those organs. Foods that are subjected to excessive heat, chemical additives, gamma radiation, and other artificial processing, as are the bulk of all modern "convenience" and supermarket foods, are entirely devoid of these life-sustaining forces of nature, regardless of how many vitamins, minerals, and proteins appear on the nutritional profiles printed on the labels.

Another aspect of energy in food is enzyme energy. Enzymes are potent biochemical and bioenergetic compounds secreted by the pancreas and other glands in the body and also contained within fresh whole foods. Enzymes are unique in that they form a bridge between "essence" (biochemistry) and "energy" (bioenergetics). To produce enzymes, the body must impart a measure of its own vital energy into the molecular structure, and this enzyme energy is utilized in virtually every vital function in the human system. When a person's diet consists entirely of enzyme-dead foods, the body must invest a lot of energy to produce enzymes to digest and process this inert dietary bulk, resulting in a net depletion of energy that robs other vital systems of the body, particularly the immune response, of the enzyme power they require to function properly. By consuming foods that are rich in enzymes, the digestive enzyme burden on the human system is relieved, freeing human energy for use in other parts of the body.

The late Edward Howell, America's leading authority on enzymes, attributes most degenerative diseases to a critical lack of active enzymes in modern diets. According to his studies, "Evidence indicates that cooked, enzyme-free diets contribute to a pathological over-enlargement of the pituitary gland, which regulates the other glands." When asked about Dr. Howell's observations regarding enzymes and energy, Master Luo Teh-hsiou, a Taoist practitioner in Taiwan, remarked:

> This energy contained in enzymes is *chee* at work in the human body, and it is contained only in fresh, unprocessed foods. Whenever you eat inert foods devoid of the *chee*-power of enzymes, your body is robbed of vital energy in order to digest and metabolize the stagnant food in your system, and this causes a constant drain of energy from the body.

The traditional Chinese diet is rich in two types of enzyme-active foods: fresh raw foods, particularly high-calorie fruits such as bananas and mangos; and foods fermented with *Aspergillus* plant enzymes, such as tofu (bean curd) and miso (fermented barley, rice, or soybean paste). All fermented roots are rich in digestive and other enzymes, and they compensate for the enzymes lost in food because of heat in cooking. When you consider the fact that over one hundred thousand different enzyme systems have been identified in operation within the human system, the importance of consuming foods rich in enzymes becomes apparent.

Another traditional Chinese method of enriching the enzyme-energy content of normally difficult-to-digest foods such as grains, seeds, and legumes is germination and sprouting. Dr. Cousens writes in *The Rainbow Diet*:

Germinating and sprouting increases the enzyme content by 6 to 20 times. Plant hormones are also activated . . . and there is a tremendous increase in metabolic activity. Starches are broken down into simple sugars, proteins are predigested into easily assimilated free amino acids, and fats are broken down into soluble fatty acids. . . . Vitamin B6 is increased by 500 percent, B5 by 200 percent, B2 by 1,300 percent, biotin by 50 percent, and folic acid by 600 percent. These biogenic foods have the capacity to generate a totally new organism. It is the life force of these foods which is transferred to people and aids their healing and regeneration.

Besides the quality of the foods you eat and how you combine them, another crucial aspect of diet and nutrition in health therapy is the way you actually eat your food. To fully extract both vital energy and nutritional essence from food, it is important to eat and drink very slowly and to deliberately savor all the constituent flavors. The Five Flavors in food are manifestations of the Five Elemental Energies of nature, and much of this energy can only be absorbed through the mucous membranes in the mouth and olfactory receptors in the sinus cavities. If you simply wolf down your food and gulp down your drinks, as so many people do these days, you miss out on the most subtle volatile energies contained in the food and beverages you consume, because the stomach is not equipped to assimilate them. Gandhi, who was a famous faster and a highly adept dietician, suggested, "Drink your food and eat your beverages," by which he meant that food should be chewed and well mixed with salivary juices until it becomes fully fluid, and beverages should be drunk as slowly as solid food is eaten.

Eating slowly not only ensures full assimilation of volatile food energy, it also ensures proper digestion of solid nutrients in the stomach, particularly carbohydrates, which must be fully ensalivated and predigested with an alkaline salivary enzyme called ptyalin to be properly digested in the stomach. All sorts of digestive distress can often be fully corrected simply by following this one rule: eat slowly, chew thoroughly, and pre-digest in the mouth before swallowing.

Undereating rather than overeating is another important factor in the Tao of diet and nutrition. All Taoist masters and traditional Chinese doctors advise their students and patients to eat *chi-ba fen bao*, which means "70 to 80 percent full." Overeating overloads the digestive system and often results in a net loss of energy rather than a gain because of the burden it puts on the digestive organs, particularly the digestive enzyme glands, such as the pancreas. Eating less than a full belly of food saves a lot of vital energy, slows the aging process, and therefore prolongs life, and this is a scientifically proven fact. Experiments conducted by Clive McCay at Cornell University have shown that the lives of rats are doubled when their food intake is reduced by half. The Venetian nobleman Luigi Cornaro (1464–1566) extended his life to one hundred and two years by cutting his intake of food down to 12 ounces per day after almost dying of obesity in his mid-forties, then further reducing it to 8 ounces per day at the age of seventy-eight. The famous centenarian peoples of Russia, Turkestan, and northern Pakistan, such as the Hunzus, consume less than 50 percent of the calories eaten daily by Americans and less than half the protein. An old Chinese proverb states, "The food that you leave on the table after a good meal does you more good than what you eat." It is as simple as that: by cutting down the quantity of food you consume daily by up to half and upgrading the quality of everything you do eat, you can greatly prolong your lifespan, particularly if you also practice periodic therapeutic fasting as part of your dietary regimen.

Eating nothing at all—fasting—is one of the most important and remarkably effective dietary therapies of all. Fasting has been practiced to purge the bowels of accumulated toxic wastes and purify the body's tissues for thousands of years in both Eastern and Western traditions, but modern medicine has entirely eliminated this marvelous healing regimen from contemporary medical practice. As a means of ridding the body of toxic residues and regenerating tissue, fasting is unparalleled by any other form of therapy. Centuries ago, the Chinese physician Chai Yu-hua wrote, "Purging the bowels eliminates the source of poisons, thereby permitting blood and energy to regenerate naturally. By cleaning the bowels we repair the body." The American naturopath Norman Walker, who lived to the age of 116 by keeping his bowels clean, wrote:

> The elimination of undigested food and other waste products is equally as important as the proper digestion and assimilation of food. . . . The very best diets can be no better than the very worst if the sewage system of the colon is clogged with a collection of waste and corruption.

Even the United States Health Service has admitted that "over 90 percent" of Americans have chronically clogged colons. The famous American faster and colonic therapist V. E. Irons puts the figure closer to 98 percent. "About the only place you see a normal healthy colon today," he once observed, "is in an anatomy book!"

Fasting is the only way to fully purge the bowels of impacted toxic wastes, purify the bloodstream and all the internal organs and glands, regenerate tissue growth throughout the system, and significantly prolong the life of the entire organism. When you fast, all your enzyme reserves, including the tremendous proportion normally preoccupied with digestive duty, enter into general circulation throughout the system and embark on a "search and destroy" mission to eliminate toxic residues, precancerous cells, newly formed tumors, accumulated chemicals, heavy metals, and other poisons from every organ, tissue, and cell in the body, and this incomparable natural healing mechanism, which all animals practice instinctively when sick, operates *only* when the body is taken entirely off its normal digestive and assimilative mode.

The Sung dynasty physician Chang Tsung-cheng used fasting and colonic cleansing therapy to cure his patients of dozens of seemingly unrelated symptoms, including respiratory ailments, chronic constipation and indigestion, headaches and fevers, arthritis and rheumatism, as well as mental and emotional disturbances. In Russia, where fasting is known as the "hunger cure," Yuri Nikolayev of the Moscow Research Institute of Psychiatry reported in 1972 that he had successfully cured over seven thousand hard-core mental patients of virtually every known form of mental disorder, including schizophrenia and psychosis. Married couples who have been childless for up to twenty years because of what their doctors told them was "infertility" have often reported their first pregnancies and childbirths after embarking on an internal cleansing program of fasting and colonic irrigation to eliminate accumulated toxic wastes from their systems.

In traditional Chinese medicine, diet and nutrition remain important pillars of health and longevity and are regarded as crucial adjuncts to all branches of medical therapy. To benefit from proper diet and nutrition, however, it is absolutely essential to first purge the entire system of accumulated wastes and purify the bloodstream; then embark on a dietary program that includes fresh, wholesome foods specifically selected to suit individual constitutional requirements; to combine food properly at all meals; to eat slowly; and to take food in moderate, measured doses, just like any other medicine.

8

Acupuncture and Moxibustion

ACUPUNCTURE AND MOXIBUSTION are ancient forms of therapy that are unique to traditional Chinese medicine and work directly with the human energy system. Traditional European, Ayurvedic, Native American, and other medical systems all practice some form of herbology, diet and nutrition, fasting, massage, breathing, and exercise as therapies for human health, but only China developed acupuncture and moxibustion, which are usually referred to together as a single branch of therapy with the traditional term *jen-jiou*, literally "needle and moxa." Both methods are applied to vital energy points (*hsueh*) located along the meridian system, and both operate by influencing the currents of electromagnetic energies that flow through the channels. These altered energy currents then carry the therapeutic effects to the targeted internal organs and tissues, balancing and regulating their functions.

According to traditional lore, acupuncture was first discovered as a result of arrow wounds suffered by soldiers on the battlefields of ancient China. Sometimes a soldier with an arrowhead embedded in his leg or arm would report the sudden disappearance of long-standing symptoms in other parts of his body, such as headaches or digestive disorders. Before long, Chinese doctors had mapped out a series of points on the surface of the body that, when pressed or punctured with crude stone implements, would have specific therapeutic effects on various other areas of the body, including internal organs, the bloodstream, the nervous system, and the muscle tissues of the limbs.

At first, sharp, flat stones called *bian* were used to press or superficially prick certain points on the surface of the body to treat various internal diseases known to respond to pressure at those points. Later, the stones were sharpened to make crude stone needles (*bian jen*) for deeper penetration. Slivers of bone and bamboo were also used for this purpose.

With the invention of metallurgy, various types of needles were fashioned from copper, iron, bronze, silver, and gold, enabling physicians to design various specifically shaped needles for different therapeutic purposes. By the second century BCE, nine kinds of needles had been developed for medical use in acupuncture, and these were recorded in the *Yellow Emperor's Classic of Internal Medicine* as follows:

Arrowhead needle: head shaped like an arrow, large and sharp, suitable for superficial pricking

Round needle: a shaft like a column, with a head rounded like an egg, used mainly for massaging the points

Blunt needle: a thick shaft and a blunt head, used for pressing on points

Triangular needle: a round shaft with a very sharp triangular-edged head, employed to cause bleeding at various points, especially on fingers and toes

Sword needle: with sharp cutting edges on both sides of the shaft, like a sword, used to make incisions for draining pus

Sharp round needle: a thick shaft with a sharp round head, used to perform fast, superficial pricking on points

Filiform needle: a shaft that is thin as a hair, with a small, sharp point; this type is most extensively used in acupuncture therapy

Long needle: a shaft about 20 cm. in length, used for deep penetration of thick tissues, such as muscle and body cavities

Large needle: a thick shaft with a rounded head, used mainly for
applying deep pressure to joints

Moxibustion is said to have been discovered even earlier than acupuncture, when people on the steppes of northern China huddled
around campfires to keep warm. They soon discovered that the heat
from the fire, besides warming their bodies, also relieved particular
pains in various parts. At first, various types of leaves, twigs, and
grasses were used, as well as glowing charcoal and bamboo embers,
but after long years of trial-and-error experimentation, it was discovered that moxa leaves (*Artemisia chinensis*) provided the most effective therapeutic benefits, particularly moxa leaves that had been
aged prior to use in moxibustion. The *Book of Mencius* (*Meng Tze*),
written during the third to fourth centuries BCE, notes, "Search out
moxa leaves that have been kept for three years to treat diseases that
have lingered for seven years." Aged moxa burns more evenly and
mildly than freshly picked leaves, and its radiant heat penetrates
more deeply into tissues. According to the master Ming dynasty
herbalist Li Shih-chen, author of the definitive Chinese materia
medica, moxibustion is particularly effective for "warming the
spleen and stomach and dispelling cold and damp." Recent studies
have shown that certain volatile oils contained in moxa leaves also
have bacteriostatic properties.

Today, moxibustion employs a sort of cigar made from tightly
rolled moxa leaves wrapped in paper. The moxa stick is lit, and the
glowing end is held over the vital point to be treated, close to but
not touching the skin, so that heat from the glowing tip radiates the
energy of the burning herb through the surface and into the point,
from where the effects travel along the affected meridians and enter
the targeted organs and tissues. An alternative form of moxibustion
involves piling a pyramid of the powdered herb on top of the point,

then igniting the top and letting it burn slowly down toward the skin, brushing away the ashes before the coal reaches the surface.

The oldest extant book devoted exclusively to acupuncture and moxibustion is A *Classic of Acupuncture and Moxibustion* (*Jen jiou jia yi jing*), written by Huangfu Mi (215–282 CE). This book records 649 vital points used in treatment and describes the various different techniques employed in clinical application. In the year 1026, during the early Sung dynasty, Wang Wei-yi compiled his famous treatise *New Illustrated Manual on the Points for Acupuncture and Moxibustion on the Bronze Man* (*Hsin tie tung ren yu hsueh jen jiou tu jing*), and in 1027 he ordered two life-sized bronze figures to be cast, illustrating and labeling all the known vital points on the human body. One of these bronzes was kept in the imperial palace, for in those days acupuncture was an esoteric skill often cultivated by aristocratic gentlemen, not only doctors, and many Chinese emperors were well known for their interest and accomplished skills in this field. The Bronze Man became a standard reference for acupuncture points for many centuries thereafter, and copies of it were cast and kept in medical academies and clinics throughout China, as well as neighboring countries such as Japan, Korea, and Vietnam.

The meridians and finer branch channels used in acupuncture and moxibustion form a gridlike network that constitutes a template outlining the entire human body (fig. 8). These channels, and the energy currents that run through them, compose a very real, albeit invisible, body of subtle energies that govern the functions of the physical body and all its parts. This energy body (*chee ti*) and its network of channels have been captured on film by a technique known as Kirlian photography, developed in Russia, where acupuncture and human energy have long been topics of serious scientific research. Mystics and psychics who have developed subtle vision by opening the so-called Celestial Eye that lies hidden between the brows are able to perceive the glow and influence the flow of these energies. Today there are psychic healers throughout the world who

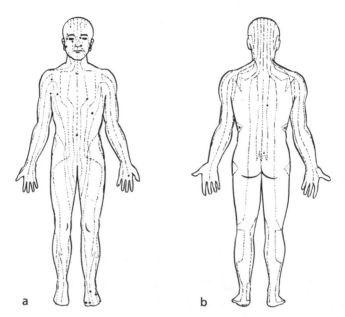

Figure 8. The meridian network of energy channels in Chinese acupuncture and acupressure, showing the yin-organ meridians (a) and yang-organ meridians (b).

diagnose and treat disease by reading the patterns and adjusting the flow of energies in the channels of the human system. The Celestial Eye is in fact a mass of magnetic cells—similar to those used as in-flight radar systems by bats and homing pigeons—located just behind the skull, between the forehead and pituitary, in all human beings, and these cells respond to the electromagnetic waves emitted by the energy systems of living organisms. The secret to awakening this power is learning how to perceive and interpret these subtle electromagnetic energy signals.

Over eight hundred vital points have been identified along the meridians of the human energy system, but in general practice, less than fifty of them are used for most common ailments. Because of the electromagnetic nature of human energy currents, metal needles inserted at vital points along the meridian network can be used to stimulate, sedate, accelerate, block, and otherwise modulate the intensity and flow of these energies, depending on which points are used and how the needles are inserted and manipulated. Since all injuries to the human body occur first on the invisible aura of energy that surrounds it, timely acupuncture therapy can prevent injuries from becoming deeply rooted somatically in the physical body. And even when an injury or disease has already become rooted, acupuncture may be used to gradually correct the associated energy imbalances responsible for the physical condition. Because the energy channels form a template that closely parallels the paths of both the nervous and blood circulatory systems, acupuncture therapy is particularly swift and effective for disorders of those systems.

Robert Becker, one of America's leading authorities on electromedicine, has done extensive research on traditional Chinese acupuncture, and his studies have conclusively established the scientific validity of acupuncture as effective medical therapy. According to Dr. Becker's work, the human body is endowed with an electromagnetic energy signal system that is far older and more fundamental in nature than the biochemically activated nervous system recognized in conventional modern medicine. It is this electromagnetic signal system that governs the body's most basic healing responses. When an injury occurs anywhere on the physical body, the electromagnetic system, not the nervous system, alerts the brain that damage has occurred and triggers the self-healing mechanisms with which all living organisms are naturally endowed. In theory, this system should enable the body not only to heal ordinary wounds, but also to regenerate entire organs and limbs that have been terminally damaged, if only the proper conditions for such a regeneration response to occur could be decoded. Based on his research in acupuncture, Dr. Becker has developed electrotherapeutic devices that help the body to reknit fractured bones; this technique has proven remarkably effective in cases where bones fail to repair themselves with conventional plaster-cast treatment.

Another important but as-yet unheralded modern spin-off from Chinese acupuncture was developed by Scottish surgeon Margaret Patterson, based on her work with a Chinese surgeon and acupuncturist in a Hong Kong hospital. The Chinese doctor, who was trained in modern Western medicine as well as traditional acupuncture, had been using electrically enhanced acupuncture to help some of his patients recover from postsurgical trauma. The treatments seemed to speed the healing of surgical wounds and also to provide considerable relief from postsurgical pain. Unknown to him, several of his patients turned out to be heroin or opium addicts, and much of their postsurgical trauma was in fact due to the intensely painful symptoms of opiate withdrawal, not surgery. Finally, some of these patients admitted their condition and reported that whenever the electrically enhanced needles were inserted into their bodies, regardless of which points were used, they experienced great relief from their withdrawal symptoms.

Working in conjunction with the results of Dr. Becker's research, Dr. Patterson determined that it was the electrical stimulus, not the needle itself, that provided the observed relief from drug withdrawal symptoms, and so she developed an electronic technique called neuro-electric therapy (NET), whereby a pulsed current is delivered to the brain from a small battery-operated device via electrodes attached to the mastoid bone area behind each ear. The key was to simulate precisely the same electromagnetic wave patterns that the brain itself produces when addicted to particular drugs, thereby triggering the same cerebral responses without the presence of the addictive drug, so that the body can detoxify itself without experiencing excruciating withdrawal symptoms. In studies conducted in Europe, Dr. Patterson's NET treatment has shown a better than 90 percent efficacy rate in curing every form of drug addiction from heroin to alcohol, without relapse, which is a far higher rate than the conventional methadone and other chemical treatments normally used today. Yet her invention remains unapproved for use in drug addiction programs in the United States and is currently employed in only a few European countries.

Acupuncture treatment for drug addiction has been practiced with remarkable success in major urban centers of the United States since the mid-1970s. At the Lincoln Hospital in the South Bronx of New York City, up to 250 addicts per day have been treated with auricular acupuncture since the program began in 1974. Resident psychiatrist Michael O. Smith reports, "In many cases, acupuncture is considered the treatment of choice. It's more highly touted all the time." Over three hundred such acupuncture detox centers are now in operation in America, and scientific studies have shown that acupuncture therapy is more effective in both the short term and long term than any other form of treatment, particularly for cocaine addiction.

One of the reasons for the success of acupuncture in the treatment of drug abuse is that acupuncture always has both psychological and physiological benefits, a phenomenon that most Western physician find difficult to understand. That is because Western medicine deals only with the body and the mind, separating them into two mutually exclusive departments, whereas Chinese medicine recognizes a third system—the human energy system—that functions as a bridge between the physical body and the psychological mind. Any treatment that works directly to balance the human energy system, such as acupuncture, balances the body as well as the mind, providing the patient with a sense of wholeness and organic integration that neither Western physiology nor psychology alone can ever achieve. As Leon Hammer, another American psychiatrist who practices acupuncture, says, "Chinese medicine doesn't distinguish between mental and physical health. Though there are about 135 points specifically for psychological manifestations, every point has some psychological effects." These combined psychic and physical effects make acupuncture a superior form of therapy in all cases where the patient's state of mind, emotional condition, and patterns of thought are closely associated with his or her physiological problems, such as in drug addiction.

Acupuncture treatment for drug addiction is based on the long-proven analgesic effects of acupuncture, which in recent years have been demonstrated to operate by virtue of acupuncture's stimulation of endorphin secretion in the brain. Endorphins are potent biochemical compounds produced naturally by the brain, and some of them are two hundred times more powerful than morphine. Unfortunately, the brain normally secretes endorphins only in emergencies, such as a sudden traumatic wound or during childbirth in women, or else during brief moments of emotional elation. Acupuncture, by stimulating the electromagnetic energy currents of the brain, which in turn govern the body's innate healing mechanisms, naturally promotes secretions of endorphins, because these pain-relieving biochemicals are intimately involved in the healing process. When enhanced with a properly pulsed electric current, the release of endorphins is even further increased. Because of this mechanism, the major clinical use of acupuncture in Western medical practice today is for analgesic relief of chronic pain. Numerous Western scientific studies have shown analgesic acupuncture to be 55 to 85 percent effective in providing real relief from chronic pain in all patients tested, which compares favorably with the 70 percent efficacy rate achieved with morphine and other chemical therapy in similar cases. The analgesic power of acupuncture is also what makes it such an effective therapy for addictive drug withdrawal.

In traditional Chinese practice there are many other therapeutic uses of acupuncture in human health care, although few Western physicians have bothered to explore them, mainly because of conceptual gaps regarding the nature of the human system. Acupuncture is routinely used in Chinese clinics to stimulate sluggish organs, sedate overactive ones, move slow bowels, reduce high blood pressure, cure insomnia and other nervous disorders, promote fertility, regulate menstrual cycles, and much more. All these applications are based on the idea that every organ, gland, and tissue in the body is governed by a network of major meridians and minor branch channels that regulate their functions by conducting the currents of vital energy on which they depend. The vital functions may therefore be therapeutically influenced by stimulating various points along the meridian network in particular ways with needles and electric currents.

One of the most interesting recent developments for acupuncture is its use as anesthesia in major surgical operations. During the 1950s, doctors in China began using long, deep-penetrating needles to achieve a sufficient state of anesthesia to perform abdominal, brain, and heart surgery. Indeed, it was this particular use of acupuncture that first brought traditional Chinese medicine to the general attention of Americans, when *New York Times* journalist James Reston underwent an emergency appendectomy under acupuncture anesthesia in Peking, while covering President Nixon's visit to China. The advantages here are obvious: not only does acupuncture anesthesia permit the patient to remain conscious, it also eliminates the long, difficult hangover and recovery period experienced by patients who undergo conventional chemical anesthesia, the effects of which are usually far more traumatic to the human system than the surgical procedure itself.

Today, scientific research continues to find more clinical applications for this traditional Chinese therapy. The English physician Felix Mann, whose books are listed in the bibliography, has been instrumental in bringing the therapeutic techniques of classical Chinese acupuncture to the attention of the Western medical community in terminology its members can understand. Bjorn Nordenstrom of the Karolinska Institute in Stockholm, has used electrically enhanced acupuncture to shrink malignant cancer tumors by inserting needles directly into the patients' tumors. The enhanced electrical field kills cancerous cells without harming healthy cells, and the pulsed energy currents help draw healing blood, energy, and immune factors to the diseased tissues to repair the damage caused by the cancerous cells.

People who have never experienced acupuncture therapy often hesitate to try it because they associate needles with the pain of getting Western-style injections or blood tests, or else because they worry about getting infected with viruses such as hepatitis B or HIV. The latter fear has become groundless owing to the current practice throughout the world of using only disposable needles in clinical acupuncture treatments. As for pain, not only is acupuncture itself quite painless, it actually provides immediate relief from chronic aches and pains throughout the entire body, while also giving the patient an integrated sense of tranquility and well-being, plus a soothing dose of endorphin secretion in the brain.

After being swiftly inserted, the needle is twirled in either direction or both directions, depending on the effect to be achieved, until a tight, tingling sensation, or a heavy numbness, is felt in the tissue just below the surface where the needle is inserted. This feeling indicates that energy is present and moving there. It is called *deh chee*, "to obtain energy," a sign that the therapy is taking effect. Acupuncture is also a very good way to get a firsthand experience for how energy feels and flows through the body via the meridian system, and this experience is useful for those who also wish to practice *chee-gung* and internal energy meditation.

As more and more Westerners choose to be trained in traditional Chinese rather than conventional Western medical sciences, both the classical and modern adaptions of acupuncture therapy, as well as moxibustion, are becoming generally available as viable alternative therapies to patients throughout the Western world. Acupuncture is currently the only traditional Chinese therapy that many medical insurance companies are now willing to cover in their health insurance policies in the U.S., and this development is rapidly bringing this branch of Chinese medicine firmly into the mainstream of modern American medical practice. Among the many conditions for which acupuncture may be effectively applied as medical therapy, the World Health Organization currently lists the following:

colds and flu
bronchitis and asthma
hay fever and sinusitis
high blood pressure
diabetes and hypoglycemia
constipation and hemorrhoids
ulcers and colon infections
indigestion and diarrhea
arthritis and bursitis
sciatica and tendinitis
headache and neuralgia
acne and eczema
stroke and paralysis
herpes
anxiety and stress
depression
insomnia
deafness and tinnitus
earaches and eye problems
impotence and infertility
premenstrual syndrome (PMS) and
    pelvic inflammatory disease (PID)
morning sickness and cramps
menstrual disorders

If a stitch in time saves nine in human health, then the acupuncture needle is an instrument that can help reweave the threads of energy in the complex tapestry of the human energy system whenever the wear and tear of life dishevels its normal woof and wrap.

9

Acupressure and Massage

ACUPRESSURE AND MASSAGE constitute the physical therapy branch of the Chinese healing arts, although like all Chinese therapies, they also have a direct impact on the human energy system as well as the mind. Acupressure involves the application of deep finger pressure to the same vital points used in acupuncture, whereas other massage techniques focus primarily on the joints, nerves, and spine, particularly the four branch channels of the bladder meridian that run parallel to the spinal cord from coccyx to neck.

Acupressure (*dian hsueh*) is the forerunner to the internationally known Japanese technique called shiatsu and has basically the same therapeutic effects as acupuncture, particularly when performed by an accomplished master who has developed the ability to transfer energy from his or her own body directly into the patient's system by pressing thumb or fingertips into the patient's vital points, while practicing internal *chee-gung*. Acupressure is used to relieve acute symptoms when needles and a clinic are not available, or when the patient is excessively sensitive to the more invasive needling techniques of acupuncture. Either the tips or the knuckles of the index and/or middle finger, and sometimes the thumb, are pressed deeply into the points selected for treatment, with sufficient pressure to achieve a therapeutic level of stimulation, but without causing the patient excessive pain. Because any point connected to an ailing organ will be especially sensitive to pressure, it is usually quite easy to find the precise location of the points required for treatment simply by observing the patient's reactions to pressure applied there. Once the point has been located and pressed, a rotating pressure is applied for a period of 10 to 15 seconds, released, then repeated as often as the therapist feels is required to achieve results.

Tui na ("push and rub") massage is usually performed with the ball of the thumb and is used to relieve arthritic and rheumatic pains in joints, activate sluggish blood circulation in muscles and other tissues, restore weak or damaged nerves, and tone the spine and spinal channels. The thumb is pushed firmly into the tissue to be treated, rubbed strongly in a circular pattern a few times, relaxed, then repeated. This therapy is applied continuously and rhythmically for periods of 20 to 30 minutes, gradually covering the entire area of treatment, such as the shoulder down to the wrist, waist down to the ankle, or entire length of the spine from neck to coccyx. In addition to its local effects, *tui na* massage has manifold therapeutic benefits for the patient's whole system: it stimulates circulation of blood and energy throughout the body, activates and drains the lymph, eliminates stagnation and toxic residues from the organs, tones the muscles, tendons, and ligaments, and enhances nerve functions. It is one of the best of all possible therapies in cases of paralysis due to stroke or injuries to the spinal cord. Spinal vertebrae that have slipped out of place respond very well to "push and rub" massage, which gradually softens the exposed cartilage and pushes it back into place between the disks, eliminating the need for surgery.

Tui na therapists pay particular attention to the four parallel channels of the bladder meridian that run along the spine, two on each side. Because of their close proximity to the spinal cord and all the autonomous nerve circuits that branch out from it, massaging these meridians and the surrounding tissues stimulates all the autonomous vital functions of the body and relaxes the muscular tension that so often blocks these nerve centers. In this age of chronic stress and hyperactivity, the muscles along the spine are usually frozen in a state of stiffness and tension, a condition that causes sustained hyperfunction of the sympathetic "action" circuit of the autonomous nervous system, also known as the "fight or flight" response. In this condition, the entire body remains in a perpetual state of alert, draining the whole system of energy and blocking such basic vital functions as digestion and immune response. Rest, restoration, and the healing response can occur only when the autonomous nervous system is switched over to the calming parasympathetic mode, and that happens only when the whole body, particularly the spine, is completely relaxed and the breath is deep and slow. By using rotating digital pressure to relax, loosen, limber, and realign the muscles, nerves, and vertebrae along the spine, the therapist induces a total relaxation of the whole body, including the internal organs, allowing the system to switch naturally over to the restorative healing circuit of the parasympathetic branch. It usually takes ten to fifteen minutes of treatment for spinal *tui na* massage to take effect, and its benefits can be clearly felt on all three levels of body, breath, and mind. Therefore, to induce this healing state of total relaxation, all Chinese massage treatments, regardless of the specific problem involved, usually include a preliminary period of spinal channel massage.

A method sometimes employed in conjuction with *tui na* therapy is cupping (*ba guan*), a form of therapy unique to traditional Chinese medicine. Either glass or bamboo cups are splashed with alcohol and quickly fired to create a vacuum inside, then firmly pressed to the area of the body to be treated. The flesh beneath the sealed rim immediately swells up into the cup because of vacuum pressure, drawing out excess damp, wind, or heat energies, and relieving tissue congestion. This method is particularly effective for acute congestion in the chest, painful joints, backache, and rheumatism, and may be applied to virtually any flat surface of the body.

Tui na techniques are also applied to the soles of the feet in a specialized branch of Chinese foot massage known in Western terminology as reflexology. Perhaps no other branch of Chinese medicine has met with as much skepticism by the Western medical community as foot massage, but anyone who has experienced its benefits can testify to its efficacy. Six of the twelve major organ-energy meridians have terminals in the feet—spleen, liver, kidneys, stomach, bladder, and gallbladder—and the major branches of the autonomous nervous system also have roots here. Therefore, by massaging particular points on the feet connected with those meridians and nerves, the therapist achieves a strong stimulation of the related internal organs and tissues of the body.

According to traditional Chinese medicine, if the feet are cramped and misshapen, as is so often the case these days because of tight, unnaturally shaped shoes and hard pavements, the associated internal organs will also be cramped and their functions inhibited. For example, chronically cramped feet are regarded as one of the major causes of impotence in men and menstrual disorders in women, owing to the obstructed flow of energy to the sexual organs and glands caused by such cramping.

Besides using their thumbs, therapists sometimes employ their knuckles or even a blunt stick to achieve deeper penetration for maximum therapeutic efficacy. After their first serious deep-tissue foot massage, many patients report an abundant excretion of very dark, sharply odorous urine, as the kidneys and bladder work to eliminate the accumulated toxins loosened and released from the internal organs and tissues as a result of the stimulation of nerve and meridian terminals in the feet.

Another specialized branch of Chinese massage therapy is head and neck massage. In a general body massage, the head and neck are usually worked on first, before the spine, to soothe the brain and central nervous system, which not only relaxes the body but also calms the patient's mind. Establishing a calm, relaxed state in the patient, both physically and mentally, is a prerequisite for the therapeutic success of any subsequent massage treatment on other parts of the body. The nerves and muscles of the neck are particularly prone to chronic tension, which causes the whole body to remain in stiff, tight condition, and this counteracts the benefits of massage therapy. These tissues must therefore be relaxed first, before other parts of the body are treated. Many important energy gates are also located on the head, especially the face, and by massaging these points at the beginning of a treatment, the associated internal organs are relaxed and the flow of energy throughout the meridian network is stimulated and balanced.

Deep-tissue massage is also applied directly to the internal organs (*nei dzang*) of the abdominal cavity to drive out accumulated toxins, release obstructions, clear stagnation, and stimulate circulation of blood and energy to the organ tissues. This form of massage employs strong pressure from the index and middle fingers, which dig deeply into the abdominal cavity to massage the targeted organs, activate their vital functions, tone their tissues, and, in the case of prolapsed organs, gradually to restore the organs to their normal shapes and locations in the abdomen. When performed by a master therapist who has developed the ability to project energy (*yun chee*) through his or her fingers, the technique is called *chee nei-dzang*, and it can be applied to correct many chronic conditions of the internal organs, including liver dysfunction, indigestion, swollen pancreas, sluggish bowels, gas, bloating, and water retention.

Another specialized branch of Chinese therapeutic massage is devoted entirely to the health care of children. Pediatric massage (*hsiao er tui na*) has a long history in the Chinese medical tradition, and it has always been an important method of responding to common childhood ailments as well as providing general preventive health care for children. Pediatric massage techniques were mentioned by

Sun Ssu-miao in his book *Precious Recipes*, written during the early Tang dynasty, and several important medical treatises devoted exclusively to massage therapy for children appeared during the Sung, Ming, and Ching dynasties.

The primary rationale for using *tui na* massage and acupressure on children, rather than acupuncture or herbal treatments, is that children's energy systems are highly responsive to manual pressure, with few of the physical or psychic barriers that often obstruct energy in adult systems, and therefore children require less intrusive techniques than adults. Children generally recoil from treatment with needles and bitter herbs, while responding well to the soothing, comforting touch of physical massage therapy. Furthermore, because the internal organs in infants and young children are still in the process of development, their meridians and points do not conform to the same patterns as those of adults, making it difficult to pinpoint the precise spots associated with particular organs. Instead, the entire area around a particular organ-energy meridian or vital point is gently massaged with rotary pressure, ensuring stimulation of the target organ system. Various oils such as sesame and almond, or aromatic balms, are often used to enhance the soothing effects of the treatment. There are 170 points used in pediatric massage and acupressure, and over half of them are specific to children's bodies. Because of the quick responsiveness of children's energy, acupressure usually achieves the same results in children that acupuncture does in adults, allowing full therapeutic effects to be achieved without alienating the child with the invasiveness of needles.

In traditional Chinese households, women learn from their mothers how to massage their infants and children as a means of general preventive health care and also to cure common childhood problems such as constipation, diarrhea, poor appetite, colds and fevers, teething, and vomiting. In addition, massage is applied to the joints, ligaments, and muscles to enhance circulation and promote proper growth of bones. It is also used to soothe hyperactive children to sleep at night. Pediatric massage, which is easy to learn and safe to practice at home, could make a big difference to the health of infants and children in the West, where childhood ailments are becoming ever more frequent and severe.

In addition to massage performed by professional doctors and physical therapists, there is also a long tradition of therapeutic self-massage in Chinese medicine. Almost all Chinese know how to press various vital energy points to achieve specific therapeutic effects for various conditions, and how to stimulate the flow of energy through their bodies and activate vital functions by massaging their own meridians. Some of the most basic and effective techniques for self-application of acupressure and massage are briefly described below.

Self-acupressure

Use the tip or knuckle of the index or middle finger, or ball of the thumb, to firmly press the following points for the conditions indicated. Press until a dull ache is felt below the surface, indicating that you have "obtained the energy," then rub with a tight rotary motion for 3 to 5 seconds, release, and repeat as often as desired.

> *Ho gu* (Valley of Harmony): Located on the lower inside corner of the back of the hand, in the cleft between the base of the thumb and forefinger, in the V about one inch below the base of the index finger. Used for relief of headaches, toothaches, and facial twitches, sore and swollen throat, and to counteract mental fatigue.
>
> *Tai chung* (Supreme Thruster): Located on top of the foot, between the bones connected to the big and second toes, about one inch from the base of those toes. For all liver ailments, including hangovers, and related headaches, dizziness, blurry vision, bloodshot eyes, high blood pressure, and nausea.
>
> *San yin jiao* (Triple Yin Crossing): Located on the inside of the calf, a hand-width up from the ankle, just behind the calf bone.

Effective for all disorders of the male and female reproductive
organs, and for stimulating sexual energy.

Nei guan (Inner Gate): On the inside of the wrist, between the
two main tendons, two finger-widths from the base of the hand.
Good for headache, insommia, epilepsy, heart palpitation, and
cardiac pain.

Yung chuan (Bubbling Spring): In the center of the ball of the
foot, about three finger-widths from the base of the middle toe.
For fainting, fright, and anxiety, hypertension, and insomnia.

Ren jung (Human Center): In the center of the depression above
the upper lip. Used for fainting, dizziness, and delirium, to stop
sneezing, and to stimulate cerebral energy.

Self-massage

Use the palms of the hands as well as the balls of the fingers and
thumbs, depending on the surface, to massage the various areas of
the body indicated below, using either a rotary rubbing or a straight
wiping motion. Before massaging each area, rub the palms and fingers briskly together until they get warm, to bring energy to the
hands and increase their polarity. Recharge the palms in this manner
between each section of the massage. Each area should be rubbed or
wiped 12 to 36 times. The following routine consitutes a general self-
massage for the whole body; the steps should be done in the order
given. It may be performed sitting on the edge of a stool or chair.

Head and neck: Use the index and middle fingers to rub circles
around the eyes, along the rims of the sockets. Next, rub down
both sides of the nose bridge, from the inside corners of the
eyes to the base of the nostrils. Place the center of the palms
on the closed eyes and rub in small circles, then do the same
on the ears. Clasp the fingers behind the head and use the
thumbs to deeply massage the cords on either side of the neck
vertebrae. Raise the head and use the palms of both hands to
alternately wipe down the whole throat and thyroid glands.

Chest: Place the centers of the palms on the nipples and rub the chest in circles. Use the palms to wipe the rib cage outward from the sternum to the sides. Use the fingers and thumb of one hand to reach across to the opposite armpit and grasp the tendons and muscles connecting the shoulder and the chest, then squeeze and rub vigorously; repeat on the other side. Use the palm of one hand to wipe down the rib cage on the opposite side, from the armpit down to the waist; repeat on the other side.

Abdomen: Use both palms to rub large circles around the abdomen, following the path of the colon from the appendix up, around, and down to the rectum. Place the center of one palm on the navel, place the other palm on top of it, and rub around in tight circles, in both directions.

Waist and lower back: Place the palms on the kidneys and wipe down to the buttocks. Place the V formed by the index fingers and thumbs on the hip bones, press inward, then rub down toward the crotch.

Thigh: Grasp the thigh muscles between the thumb and fingers and squeeze vigorously, working down toward the knees. Slap the outsides of the thighs with open palms, working down from the hips to the knees.

Knees: Massage around the rims of the kneecaps with the thumbs and fingers; rotate the kneecaps with the centers of the palms.

Calves: Cross one calf across the other knee, then use the thumbs and fingers of both hands to grasp the calf muscle and knead vigorously, working down from the knees to the ankles.

Ankles: Grasp the ankle with one hand and use the other hand to rotate the entire foot in circles on the ankle joint.

Feet: Press the *tai chung* point on the top of the feet, between the bones of the large and second toes, then use thumb pressure to rub down the entire length of the depressions between all the bones on the tops of the feet. Press the *yung chuan* points in the center of the balls of the feet and rub in tight circles. Grasp each toe and knead it vigorously.

Arms: Use the palm to wipe down the entire length of the arm from the shoulder to the wrist, then grasp the forearm muscle between the fingers and thumb and squeeze vigorously, working down from the elbow to the wrists.

Hands: Press the thumb into the *lao gung* point in the center of the palm and place the index and middle fingers on top of the hand, then squeeze deeply. Press the *ho gu* point with the thumb (see p. 116). Use the thumb and index finger to grasp each finger at its base, then knead vigorously outward to the tips.

A unique type of self-massage in Chinese tradition is the sexual self-massage used by Taoist adepts to cultivate internal energy for transformation into spiritual vitality. Known as Solo Cultivation (*dan hsiou*), in contrast to the Dual Cultivation (*shuang hsiou*) of sexual yoga practiced with a partner, it involves using the palms of the hands to massage the testicles in men and the breasts in women, employing the *lao gung* energy point in the center of the palms. Prior to performing this massage, the palms are briskly rubbed together to draw energy into them and enhance their polarity, to increase the effects of the massage. The purpose of this form of massage is certainly not to achieve sexual pleasure, but rather to stimulate secretions of essential hormones in the sexual glands. The energy harvested from this vital essence is called *jing-chee* (Essential Energy) and is drawn into general circulation via the meridians using deep breathing and visualization techniques. It is an effective way to cultivate internal energy, to balance yin and yang, and to stimulate the endocrine system.

Of all the branches of traditional Chinese therapy, acupressure and massage are probably the easiest for most people to learn how to apply to themselves and others as a means for general preventive health care, for the relief of chronic physical discomforts, and as a palliative for many common ailments. One of the best practical manuals for learning Chinese therapeutic massage techniques is Yang Jwing-ming's comprehensive text and illustrated guide, *Chinese Qigong Massage* (listed in the bibliography). Unlike acupuncture and herbal therapy, which require a professional hand, or *chee gung* and meditation, which take some time to learn and must be practiced daily, acupressure and massage can be performed anytime, anywhere, by anyone.

10

Chee-gung and Exercise

CHEE-GUNG IS AN ANCIENT Chinese method of self-health care and life extension that combines slow rhythmic movements of the body with deep abdominal breath control in a harmonious dance of life choreographed by a tranquil, meditative state of mind. Sometimes referred to by Western adepts as "moving meditation," *chee-gung* was known in ancient China as the method for eliminating disease and prolonging life. In the opinion of this writer and practitioner, Chinese *chee-gung* is by far the most profound and effective system for the self-cultivation of health and longevity ever developed.

Chee means "breath" and "air" as well as "energy," and *gung* refers to any skill that takes a lot of time and discipline to develop and great self-control to perform. Hence *chee-gung* may be translated in English as "the skill of breath and energy control." *Chee-gung* has been practiced for health and longevity since the dawn of civilization in China, and references to it appear in the earliest annals of Chinese history. It evolved first as a sort of therapeutic dance to relieve rheumatic pains and circulatory stagnation due to excessive dampness in the humid, flood-prone plains of the Yellow River in northern China, where Chinese civilization was born. An inscription found on jade tablets dating from the sixth century BCE states, "Whoever follows this method will live a long life. Whoever goes against it will die prematurely."

During the Warring States period (fifth–second centuries BCE), *chee-gung* forms were based on the movements of animals in nature, a system known as the Play of the Five Beasts *(wu chin hsi)*. In the *Collective Commentaries on Chuang Tzu*, written in the second century BCE, Cheng Yuan-lin states, "Breathing practiced together with movements resembling a bear, bird, and other animals helps move our *chee*, nourishes our bodies, and builds our spirits." The centenarian Tang dynasty physician Sun Ssu-miao extolled the health benefits of proper breathing in his landmark medical treatise *Precious Recipes*:

> When correct breathing is practiced, the myriad ailments will not occur. When breathing is depressed and strained, all sorts of diseases will arise. Those who wish to nurture their lives must first learn the correct methods of controlling breath and balancing energy. These breathing methods can cure all ailments great and small.

In addition to properly regulated breathing, the other pillar of *chee-gung* practice is soft, gently flowing physical exercise, a type of exercise known as *dao-yin* ("induce and guide"). In the fourth century BCE Confucian classic entitled *Spring and Autumn Annals*, this sort of exercise, which is unique to traditional Chinese health care, is described as follows:

> Flowing water never stagnates, and the hinges of an active door never rust. This is due to movement. The same principle applies to essence and energy. If the body does not move, essence does not flow. When essence does not flow, energy stagnates.

The famous doctor and Taoist adept Hua To, whose life spanned 100 years during the second to third centuries CE, developed a series of therapeutic *dao-yin* exercises based on the fighting postures of animals and prescribed them as a cure for arthritis, rheumatism, gastric ailments, nervous disorders, and circulatory problems. "When the blood flows unobstructed through the veins," he wrote, "illness cannot take root. This is like a door hinge that cannot rust owing to frequent use." A century later, the great Taoist alchemist and esoteric writer Ko Hung, author of the encyclopedic Taoist tome *Pao Pu Tzu* ("Embracing the Uncarved Block"), observed, "The onset of illness is a sign that *chee* is not flowing. One must exercise to unblock the myriad meridians and facilitate the free flow of *chee*."

In the fifth century CE, there appeared in China an eccentric Buddhist monk from India named Bodhidharma, known in Chinese history as Ta Mo. Bodhidharma brought with him the *pranayama* breathing exercises of Indian yoga and fused them with the *dao-yin* animal-form exercises he found in China, creating a unique style of breath control combined with physical exercise that became the basis for all subsequent schools of *chee-gung* in China. Bodhidharma wrote two books that later became the classic bibles of all forms of medical, martial, and meditative *chee-gung* practice in China as well as Japan and Korea. The first is entitled *The Tendon Changing Classic (Yi Chin Ching)* and deals mainly with stretching, loosening, and basic breathing postures. The second is *The Marrow Cleansing Classic (Hsi Sui Ching)*, which introduces the secrets of internal alchemy (*nei-gung*) and other advanced practices, such as Solo Cultivation and transformation of sexual energy for spiritual purposes. These two classics have inspired virtually every school of *chee-gung* and formed the foundation of every style of practice that developed in subsequent centuries in China, and to this day Bodhidharma, who was also the first patriarch of Chan (Zen) Buddhism, is still revered as the patron saint of all the traditional martial arts sects in China, Japan, and Korea.

The concept of *chee* remains one of the greatest stumbling blocks between the modern Western and traditional Chinese medical systems, despite the fact that modern science has conclusively established the existence of both electromagnetic and infrared light energies within the human system, thereby confirming the traditional Chinese paradigm of how *chee* operates in the human body. Scientific research at Jiao Tong University in Shanghai, employing sophisticated modern technology, has shown that human energy manifests the properties of electromagnetic currents when flowing within the meridian system, but that it takes on the properties of particle streams, similar to laser light energy, when projected out from the body through the hands of master *chee-gung* healers, who cure disease by beaming their energy into the patient's system. The penetrating power of this projected human energy exceeds that of alpha and beta rays, easily passing through wood and metal sheets, and it can travel distances of up to 150 meters without losing power.

Traditional Chinese medicine refers to the unique form of energy that animates the human system as *jeng-chee* ("True Energy"), to distinguish it from the other types of energy found in nature, such as the Five Elemental Energies of the planet and the universal free energy of the cosmos. A distinctive property of True Energy is its capacity to carry information as well as project power. The information carried by True Energy is imprinted by the human mind, and it is this information imprint that enables *chee-gung* healers to specifically pattern the energy they project into their patients' systems to suit their particular medical requirements. Studies on *chee-gung* healers in China have shown that they can modulate their energy transmissions to kill specific microbes, dissolve tumors, stimulate the heart, and so forth. These findings verify one of the most ancient axioms of Taoist internal alchemy: "Spirit commands energy, energy commands essence"—that is, the mind controls and directs energy in particular patterns in order to cause specific physiological effects in the body.

The primary purpose of practicing *chee-gung* on an individual basis is to "cultivate True Energy" (*yang jeng-chee*) for health and longevity. *Chee-gung* practice increases one's potential energy reserves and enhances the functional activity of every organ, tissue, and cell in the body. The energy is stored in an area just below and behind the navel known as the Sea of Energy (*chee-hai*), or the Elixir Field (*dan-tien*) (fig. 9). The role of the Sea of Energy in the human system is described by the Ching dynasty physician Chang Chin-chiou in his commentary on *The Yellow Emperor's Classic of Internal Medicine*:

> Man is born attached at the navel to an umbilical cord, and the navel is connected to the lower Elixir Field, which is the Sea of Energy. Thus the navel forms the Gate of Life. The fetus receives life through the opening of this gate, and the infant enters this world by its closing. Therefore, in its capacity as a spring of living energy, this region is the source of

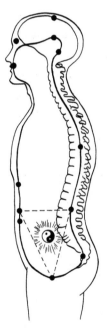

Figure 9. The Sea of Energy, or Elixir Field (dan-tien), *in the lower abdomen, where human energy is stored.*

man's well-being and his discomfort, his strength and his weakness. When the energy here is strong, the whole system is strong. When it is weak, the whole system grows weak.

The navel is where Fire and Water meet, where Yin and Yang reside. It is the sea of essence and energy, the door of life and death.

Chee-gung exercises "induce and guide" (*dao-yin*) energy to circulate to each of the vital organ-energy systems and to flow freely throughout the entire human body, enabling the body to achieve a state of enhanced vitality that protects the whole system from disease and degeneration and prolongs the life of the entire organism. The practice enlists the Three Treasures of essence, energy, and spirit in a harmonious exercise that benefits all three levels of human existence—body, breath, and mind. On the physical level, the rhythmic movements of the limbs limber the joints, tone the muscles, activate the blood, and gently massage all the internal organs and glands. On the mental level, the cerebral cortex, which normally consumes a tremendous amount of energy with its ceaseless mental chatter and discursive meanderings, is silenced and suspended, permitting internal energy to flow uninhibited throughout the system. The importance of establishing mental tranquility and an "empty" state of mind through suspension of discursive thought cannot be overstated in *chee-gung*, for mental quiescence is an absolute precondition for inducing the unobstructed flow of True Energy through the meridian system. As *The Yellow Emperor's Classic of Internal Medicine* states, "When the mind is quiescent and void, True Energy will be at your command. If one maintains a tranquil mind, the danger of disease will turn to safety."

Breath and energy, however, are the real pivots of *chee-gung* practice. When practicing *chee-gung* and *dao-yin* exercises with a tranquil mind and a relaxed, rhythmically moving body, the breath grows deep and regular, and True Energy naturally begins to flow freely through the system. Known as "running the channels" (*dzou jing-mai*), this free flow of internal energy clears stagnant *chee* from the meridians and congested blood from the organs and pumps fresh energy through all twelve vital organ-energy systems, simultaneously feeding them with freshly oxygenated blood. As another axiom of internal alchemy states, "Energy commands blood, and blood follows energy. Where energy goes, blood follows." At the same time, all the external tissues of the body, such as muscles, skin, and fascia, are also flushed with fresh blood as energy flows through the web of channels that permeates the physical body.

On another level, *chee-gung* practice literally "tunes in" the body to the prevailing pulse of the earth's frequency, a frequency known as the Schumann resonance, which vibrates at 7.8 herz (cycles/second). This is the ambient vibration of the planet, which constitutes the most important macrocosmic supersystem for the human energy system. This has been shown to be the most perfect frequency for healing and harmonizing the human energy system, for it permits the human system to resonate in perfect synchronicity with the pulse of the planet. A daily session of *chee-gung* practice therefore serves as a whole-system tune-up for the entire human organism and all its constituent organ-energy subsystems, establishing a harmonic resonance with the earth that has powerful healing and preventive-health properties.

Another unique benefit of *chee-gung* practice is that it balances the endocrine and nervous systems, bringing them into harmonic synchronicity via positive biofeedback mediated by hormones and neurotransmitters. Deep abdominal breathing, physical relaxation, and mental quietude—the three pillars of *chee-gung* practice— naturally switch the autonomous nervous system from the hyperactive sympathetic circuit over to the restorative healing mode of the parasympathetic branch. Modern urban lifestyles, which promote a constant state of stress, hyperactivity, and cerebral excitation, tend to keep the nervous system in a perpetual sympathetic mode of operation. This condition inhibits basic vital functions, weakens the immune response, and drains the whole system of energy. By practicing *chee-gung* on a daily basis, you can counteract the stressful effects of excessive sympathetic nervous response by shifting your system over to the rejuvenating, relaxing parasympathetic circuit, and this can be done any time of day, any place you wish to practice. Taoist master Luo Teh-hsiou of Taiwan describes this effect as follows:

> *Chee-gung* activates the parasympathetic circuit of the central nervous system, thereby stimulating the production of neurochemicals which cause the endocrine system to secrete hormones that enhance vitality and boost immunity. Those hormones also help sustain further production of calming parasympathetic neurochemicals. This mutual interaction continues until perfect equilibrium is established between the nervous and endocrine systems, and when that happens, the True Energy of human health and longevity is generated.

To grasp the internal dynamics of *chee-gung* and learn how to practice it properly, it is important to understand the role played by the diaphragm in deep abdominal breathing. The diaphragm is a tough but flexible muscle that separates the chest from the abdominal cavity. In deep abdominal breathing, the diaphragm descends toward the abdominal organs on inhalation and rises back into the chest cavity on exhalation, providing a vigorous massage to the organs and glands, particularly the kidneys and adrenals. It also enhances blood circulation throughout the system by virtue of the shifting pressures it creates, like a pump between chest and abdomen. Owing to laziness, congestion, emotional inhibition, stress, smoking, pollution, and other factors, modern men and women typically engage in shallow upper-chest breathing, a condition associated with the state of anxiety, rather than the deep abdominal breathing for which our systems were designed. A. Salmanoff describes the respiratory functions of the diaphragm and the benefits of its proper use in breathing:

It is the most powerful muscle in our body; it acts like a perfect force-pump, compressing the liver, the spleen, the intestines, and stimulating the whole abdominal and portal circulation.

By compressing the lymphatic and blood vessels of the abdomen, the diaphragm aids the venous circulation, from the abdomen towards the thorax.

The number of movements of the diaphragm per minute is a quarter of those of the heart. But its haemodynamic power is much greater than that of cardiac contractions because the surface of the force-pump is much greater and because its propelling power is superior to that of the heart. We have only to visualize the surface of the diaphragm to accept the fact that *it acts like another heart.*

The importance of the diaphragm's role as a "second heart" in *chee-gung* practice cannot be overemphasized, and this function may be further enhanced by a technique known as reverse abdominal breathing, or the abdominal lock, whereby the abdominal wall is drawn inward on inhalation, rather than being permitted to expand outward. This simple maneuver greatly increases the pressure within the abdominal cavity as the diaphragm descends on inhalation. The extra pressure created by the contraction of the abdominal wall during inhalation gives a strong boost to the upward flow of blood through the vena cava, a major vein that penetrates the diaphragm and draws stale blood from the abdominal organs up to the heart and lungs for replenishment with fresh oxygen. This propulsive force, which acts like a powerful suction pump, is far stronger than the propulsive force of the heart, and it boosts blood circulation throughout the entire extent of the circulatory system, taking a tremendous load off the heart with every deep abdominal breath. When you consider the fact that the brain alone is irrigated by 2,000 liters of blood per day and contains about 1,000 meters of capillaries per gram, the importance of this extra circulatory boost provided by the diaphragm becomes even more apparent, particularly for sedentary people who do a lot of cerebral work and do not get much vigorous physical exercise to stimulate circulation.

Another important maneuver in *chee-gung* practice is the anal sphincter lock, known in Chinese as *ti-gang* ("lifting the anus") and in Indian yoga as *mula bandha*. As the abdominal wall expands and is then deliberately contracted on inhalation, internal pressure in the abdominal cavity increases, and this pressure naturally tries to escape downward through the soft tissue of the pelvic floor and anus. To prevent this escape and maintain the beneficial internal pressure in the abdomen, one must gently but firmly contract and lock the anal sphincter, a maneuver that lifts the entire pelvic floor and seals in the enhanced abdominal pressure. Instead of escaping downward, the pressure is maintained inside, where it massages the internal organs, stimulates the glands, and works as a pump to boost the circulatory system.

The pelvic floor consists of a pliant web of muscles, tendons, and nerves that acts somewhat like a second diaphragm; it is known as the urogenital diaphragm. Every contraction of the anal sphincter gives a therapeutic stimulation to the sacral nerves that run through this diaphragm, activating secretions of vital hormones in the testicles and ovaries, balancing prostate and menstrual functions, promoting peristalsis in the bowels and other digestive tract functions, toning the bladder and urogenital canal, and clearing stagnant blood from the capillaries of the anus, helping prevent or cure hemorrhoids. The anal lock and pelvic lift may be practiced any time, any place, in any posture, with or without *chee-gung* breathing, and always provides excellent therapeutic benefits to the entire sacral circulation and associated functions.

Chee-gung practice begins with the lungs and deep abdominal breathing, but ultimately it trains you to breathe with your entire body and move energy directly through various energy "gates." This is accomplished by gradually shifting your internal mental focus from the flow of air in and out of the nostrils and lungs over to the flow of energy in and out of selected energy gates, such as the Celestial Eye between the eyebrows, the Medicine Palace on top of the skull, the Bubbling Spring on the soles of the feet, the Labor Palace on the palms of the hands, the Gate of Life between the kidneys, and the Confluence of Yin at the perineum. When the breath has become perfectly regulated, the mind tranquil, and the body fully relaxed, you simply shift your awareness to one of these points and breathe through it, visualizing and sensing a stream of light entering on inhalation and exiting on exhalation. A sensation of tingling, warmth, or numbness at the point selected for practice indicates that the gate has opened and energy is streaming through it. Highly advanced adepts of "body breathing" can actually suspend air and lung breathing and breathe entirely through their energy gates, drawing pure energy directly into their meridians.

The medical applications and therapeutic benefits of *chee-gung* and *dao-yin* exercises are manifold, and they are profoundly effective when properly practiced, particularly in conjunction with proper diet, tonic herbs, therapeutic massage, and other regimens. Among major health benefits are the following:

Adaptogenic: The practice of *chee-gung* adapts the entire system to deal successfully with adverse environmental conditions and sudden aberrations in external energy factors, such as inclement weather, pollution, geographical changes due to travel, stress, and so forth. It does this by internally rebalancing the human energy system to compensate for imbalances in the environment.

Digestive: Chee-gung practice stimulates the secretion of bile and digestive enzymes, activates peristalsis, massages all the digestive organs, enhances the flow of blood and energy to the abdominal organs, clears stagnation, and helps cure and prevent every sort of digestive disorder.

Circulatory: The practice of *chee-gung* boosts the circulation and distribution of blood throughout the entire system, clears stagnant blood from organs and capillaries, oxygenates the blood, regulates blood pressure, and deepens and slows the pulse.

Stress management: The practice of *chee-gung* eliminates anxiety and stress by directly counteracting their effects on the energy system. It lowers cortisone levels in the blood, reduces erratic activity in the cerebral cortex, normalizes and deepens respiratory patterns, switches the autonomic nervous system over from the fight-or-flight sympathetic mode to the relaxing, restorative parasympathetic circuit.

Emotional equlibrium: The practice of *chee-gung* fosters a state of emotional equilibrium by harmonizing the Five Elemental Energies of the organs and balancing yin and yang throughout the system. Because emotional reactions are simply "energies in motion" that have run out of control, *chee-gung* immediately reestablishes emotional equilibrium by harnessing and harmonizing those energies.

Immunity: The practice of *chee-gung* stimulates and balances endocrine secretions throughout the system, particularly in the pituitary/adrenal axis, thereby enhancing the immune response. It increases the activity of bone marrow, which produces white blood cells. It activates the psychoneuroimmunological (PNI) response by creating positive biofeedback between the neurotransmitters of the nervous system and the hormones of the endocrine system, and it engages the healing responses of the parasympathetic branch of the autonomic nervous system.

Yin-yang pH (acid-alkaline) balance: The practice of *chee-gung* maintains a healthy pH balance in the bloodstream and other tissues, eliminating the debilitating effects of chronic acidosis. Physical exercise alone acidifies blood, whereas deep breathing alone alkalizes it. *Chee-gung* breathing combined with gentle, rhythmic *dao-yin* exercise maintains proper yin-yang pH balance in the blood and other bodily fluids.

There are many schools and forms of *chee-gung* practice, ranging from the extreme "external skills" (*wai-gung*) of combative martial arts such as Shao Lin, Karate, and Tai Kwon Do, to the subtle internal alchemy (*nei-gung*) practices of Taoist meditation methods. There are therapeutic *chee-gung* techniques used in medical practice, whereby the therapist transfers his or her energy directly into the patient's system to achieve specific therapeutic effects, and there are self-care methods in which the patient practices specific exercises to heal particular systems within his or her own body. The most popular styles of *chee-gung* and *dao-yin* exercise for health and longevity involve a balanced blend of breath control and rhythmic physical exercise, meditation and martial arts, and internal alchemy and external movement; and these forms have both curative and preventive health benefits. These are the "moving meditation" styles of *chee-gung*, which you can see Chinese teachers and their students practicing in public parks and private gardens during the early hours of the morning or toward sunset—such styles as Tai Chi, Pa Kua, Hsing Yi, and Pa Tuan Chin—and virtually anyone who can stand on their own two feet can learn to perform these elegant energy exercises to keep their "waters flowing" and their "hinges active" and dance their way to health and longevity.

11
Meditation and Internal Alchemy

IN CHINESE TRADITION, besides its role in higher spiritual cultivation, meditation is also regarded as an important therapeutic practice for health and longevity. "Meditation" is a poor translation for
what the Chinese and most other Asian cultures simply refer to as
"sitting" (*da dzuo*), or in Taoist tradition "sitting still doing nothing"
(*jing dzuo wu wei*). The word *meditation* implies some sort of ab-
stract mental musing or complex spiritual exercise, whereas the real
point of sitting still doing nothing is to empty the mind entirely of
all conceptual thought, to silence the internal dialogue and simply
let the mind abide in a natural state of tranquility and silence. This
seems particularly difficult for Westerners, who feel that time not
spent doing something, even if it is only indulging in idle fantasy or
watching TV, is time wasted. Nothing could be farther from the
truth, for even a few brief minutes of genuine mental calm, with the
mind as still and clear as a mountain lake on a windless and cloudless
day, can do more to promote health and prolong life than the most
expensive medicines on the earth. As the French philosopher Blaise
Pascal observed, "All of man's misery comes from his inability to sit
quietly in a room all by himself and do nothing."

Meditation is the highest level of internal *chee-gung* practice and is referred to in esoteric Taoist terminology as "internal alchemy" (*nei-gung*). As discussed earlier, according to the Triplex Unity of the Three Treasures of essence, energy, and spirit, essence is conserved and then converted into energy; energy is stored in the Elixir Field below the navel and then raised and transformed to nurture spirit. When spirit has become clear and stable through this practice, it is then able to exercise its primordial power of command over energy, which it focuses and directs in order to exert control over essence, thereby completing the cycle of internal alchemy and restoring the entire sytem—body, energy, and mind—to its primordial state of self-perfected harmony and self-sustaining health.

While herbs and diet work directly with essence (the physical level of existence), and acupuncture and *chee-gung* work directly with energy, meditation and internal alchemy approach the human system from the highest level of spirit. By virtue of the Triplex Unity that binds body, energy, and mind into one organic system, all three levels of approach influence all three modes of existence. The ultimate goals of health and longevity, balance and harmony, are the same in all health care practices; the only difference lies in the avenue of approach into the system. From the point of view of health care, meditation is just another therapeutic means of nurturing and balancing the human energy system. In the case of meditation, healing energy is drawn directly into the system from nature and the cosmos via the body's energy gates, converted in the "cauldrons" of the body's energy centers (chakras) to produce the True Energy on which the human system depends, then distributed to the various organs, glands, and tissues through the body's network of meridians and channels. The sole precondition for this process to occur is to achieve a truly tranquil state of mental quietude and physical relaxation, a state that is mediated and maintained by smooth, rhythmically regulated breathing.

When the body is resting in a stable meditative posture, with the mind calm and silent, the human energy system becomes a vessel into which the ever-present energies of nature and the cosmos pour freely, like water into a jug. Universal free energy funnels into the human system in a spiral pattern through the Medicine Palace (*nee wan gung*) point on the crown of the head and through other gates, such as those on the palms of the hands, on the soles of the feet, between the brows, on the perineum, and along the spine. This energy constitutes a form of "free medicine" that is always available to anyone who has the patience to learn how to sit still and administer it.

Meditation, or simply "sitting still doing nothing," is the method by which the universal free energy of nature and the cosmos is "digested" and assimilated by the human energy system. This process is accomplished by virtue of the piezoelectric properties of the bones and other crystalline structures of the human body, as discussed earlier in the chapter on the human energy system. The energy that spirals into the human system from the sky and earth is invisible vibrational wave energy, and this high-frequency wave energy is "stepped down" as it passes through the various energy centers, or chakras, of the human system. It is then converted by the crystalline structures of the body into electromagnetic energy pulses, or True Energy, and fed via the meridian network to all the organs and tissues of the body. Thus meditation transforms wave energy from external sources into the type of electromagnetic energy required by the human system, just as food is transformed into energy by the digestive system on the physical level. People who practice meditation on a daily basis automatically avail themselves of a free daily dose of this pure, potent energy-medicine, recharging their biobatteries and topping off their energy tanks every day with the highest-grade energy of all, the same energy that fuels nature and the cosmos.

Another form of vibrational energy medicine that can be transformed into healing energy pulses for the human system through the practice of meditation is mantra, the sacred syllables chanted in tantric Buddhist and Hindu meditation systems. In Chinese Taoist tradition, similar effects are achieved with a series of "healing sounds" designed to tone and heal various internal organs and glands. The syllables used in mantra and healing sound practice have been specifically selected to produce beneficial therapeutic effects within the human system when chanted in a state of mental quietude and physical relaxation. Just like any other vibrational energy, these sonorous waves are transformed by the bones and crystalline tissues of the body into electromagnetic pulses by virtue of the piezoelectric effect, and these pulses of True Energy then spread and resonate throughout every tissue and cell of the body, synchronizing with the body's own internal energies in patterns that have remarkable healing properties. The therapeutic benefits of soothing music for convalescing patients, agitated animals, and growing plants have been observed in numerous scientific studies, and this same mechanism operates in vibrational mantra and healing-sound meditation.

A course in meditation is beyond the scope of this book, but basically it involves adopting a stable sitting posture, with the spine held erect, the neck straight, and the shoulders and chest relaxed. You may sit cross-legged on a cushion on the floor, on the edge of a stool or chair, or even lie down on your side on the floor or in bed. The eyes should be neither tightly shut nor wide open but kept half-lidded and unfocused, and the tip of the tongue should be lightly pressed to the palate, just behind the upper teeth, to complete the energy circuit of the Microcosmic Orbit formed by the two energy channels that run from the perineum up the spine and over the head to the palate, and from the mouth down the chest to the perineum. The breath should be even, regular, and natural, and the mind should be allowed to rest in complete tranquility by simply letting all thoughts gradually fade away and disappear, like a train passing through in the night.

One of the easiest meditation methods to learn, for health and longevity, especially for those who have never practiced before, is the system developed by Master Han Yu-mo of Taiwan and contained in his handbook *Directions for Meditational Techniques* (listed in the bibliography). Master Han's methods enable the practitioner to funnel cosmic energies into his or her system through the Medicine Palace gate on top of the head, then blend them with one's own internal energies and use the enhanced True Energy to clear obstructions from within the energy channels; fortify muscles, tendons, fascia, and bones; and heal injuries to the internal organs and glands. The clearing process often causes a rocking or swaying motion in the body, as energy surges strongly through the channels and eliminates blockages to the free flow of *chee*. This rocking motion may be enlisted and directed to cure specific ailments, such as arthritis, back pain, clogged bowels, headaches, and so forth.

Paracelsus, one the most enlightened medical masters in Western history, wrote, "The human body is vapor materialized by sunshine mixed with the life of the stars." His view of the human system as condensed energy emanating from the same universal source as the sun and stars accords remarkably with the traditional Chinese view of the human energy system and its functional interdependence with the energies of nature and the cosmos. Today, however, Parcelsus' vitalist school of thought has been totally eradicated from Western medical philosophy and practice by the chemical-mechanical paradigm promoted by modern pharmaceutical and surgical medicine.

As long as Western medicine continues to cling to its chemical-mechanical approach to human health and healing, it will continue to deprive its patients of the greatest healing power of all, the very life force that lies at the heart of the human organism and is freely available to one and all from its orginal sources in nature and the cosmos. As Deng Ming-dao wrote in *The Wandering Taoist,*

> If you want to preserve your health, attain longevity, and pierce life's mysteries, you must seal in the life force . . . and practice *chee-gung* and meditation to retain and circulate the life force that is rooted in *jing* [essence].

In order to do this, *jing* reacts with breath and becomes *chee*. *Chee* is circulated and transformed into spirit. It is spirit-energy that reaches the top.

All this can be accomplished by the simple, easy-to-practice method of "sitting still doing nothing." As an old Chinese meditation master once told his fidgety Western students, "Don't just do something—sit there!"

Annotated Bibliography

Becker, R. *The Body Electric*. New York: William Morrow, 1985.

A scientific analysis of the electromagnetic nature of the human energy system and its evolutionary development, with commentary on Chinese acupuncture, self-healing mechanisms, tissue regeneration, and other related topics.

———. *Cross Currents*. Los Angeles: Jeremy Tarcher, 1990.

An in-depth scientific discussion of the role of the electromagnetic human energy system in health and healing, including important revelations on electromagnetic pollution as a modern cause of human disease and various modes of healing with electromagnetic medicine, written by one of America's leading authorities in the field.

Beinfield, H., and E. Korngold. *Between Heaven and Earth: A Guide to Traditional Chinese Medicine*. New York: Ballantine Books, 1991.

A detailed and comprehensive guide to the philosophy and practical therapeutic branches of traditional Chinese medicine, written in a lucid style for the general Western reader. Includes many explanatory charts and schematic diagrams to illustrate basic concepts, plus chapters for practical self-analysis of constitutional types and guidelines for dietary and herbal therapy at home.

Bensky, D., and R. Barolet. *Chinese Herbal Medicine: Formulas and Strategies*. Seattle: Eastland Press, 1990.

A compilation and translation of classical Chinese resource materials regarding traditional herbal formulas and their therapeutic applications.

Blate, M. *The Natural Healer's Acupressure Handbook*. New York: Henry Holt, 1977. Falkynor Press.

A practical manual for Chinese acupressure therapy, with illustrated techniques and detailed instructions for practice at home.

Blofeld, John. *I Ching: The Book of Change*. London, Unwin: 1976.

Blofeld's translation of this ancient book of divination remains one of the clearest versions for Western readers without previous exposure to classical Chinese philosophy. It includes a foreword by Lama Govinda, excellent explanatory chapters, and numerous charts and diagrams to illustrate how the trigrams and hexagrams work.

Chang, S. T. *The Complete System of Chinese Self-Healing*. London: Thorsons, 1989.

A complete guide to traditional Chinese *chee-gung* and *dao-yin* exercises for health and longevity, including breathing techniques, body exercises, self-massage, and internal alchemy meditation, illustrated and clearly explained, with introductory chapters on theoretical foundations.

Cline, K. *Chinese Pediatric Massage: Practitioner's Reference Manual*. Portland, Wash.: Institute for Traditional Medicine, 1993.

A practical guide to traditional Chinese therapeutic massage for children, including introductory commentary on theory and clear instructions on actual techniques.

―――. *A Parent's Guide: Chinese Pediatric Massage*. Portland, Wash.: Institute for Traditional Medicine, 1993.

An illustrated manual for parents who wish to use Chinese pediatric massage for curative and preventive therapy at home.

Cousens, G. *Spiritual Nutrition and the Rainbow Diet*. San Rafael, Calif.: Cassandra Press, 1986.

An interesting and informative discussion of diet and nutrition from the perspective of human energetics, with important scientific explanations of the internal alchemy of energy transformation in the human system.

Dharmananda, S. *Chinese Herbal Therapies for Immune Disorders*. Portland, Wash.: Institute for Traditional Medicine, 1988.

Traditional Chinese herbs and formulas for enhancement of the human immune response, with an explanation of the Chinese medical view on immune deficiency disorders.

Fan, Y. L. *Chinese Pediatric Massage Therapy: A Parent's and Practitioner's Guide to the Treatment and Prevention of Childhood Diseases*. Boulder, Colo.: Blue Poppy Press, 1994.

A comprehensive guide to and practical manual on the therapeutic applications of Chinese pediatric massage therapy in the clinic and at home, with detailed instructions on various techniques.

Fratkin, J. *Chinese Classics*. Boulder, Colo.: Shya Publications, 1990.

A guide to sixty-four popular classic Chinese herbal formulas and their uses, with an alphabetical index of symptoms, a glossary of terms, and a list of suppliers.

————. *Chinese Herbal Patent Formulas*. Boulder, Colo.: Shya Publications, 1986.

A complete guide to a broad range of Chinese patent formulas, including classical formulas from China and contemporary adaptations made in America, with detailed information on indications, dosage, and ingredients, and a list of mail-order suppliers.

Hammer, L. *Dragon Rises, Red Bird Flies: Psychology and Chinese Medicine*. Barrytown, N.Y.: Station Hill Press, 1990.

A general introduction to the basic concepts of traditional Chinese medicine, focusing on their psychological and emotional aspects, written by a Western psychiatrist who uses acupuncture in his private practice; a subjective exploration of Chinese medicine, using terms and psychic symbols to which Western readers can readily relate.

Han Yu-mo. *Directions for Meditational Techniques*. Taipei: Yu Mo Publishing, 1994.

A translation by Daniel Reid and Ronald Brown of Master Han Yu-mo's illustrated manual of Taoist meditation and internal alchemy, focusing on health and longevity practices, including fundamental and advanced levels.

Hsu, H. Y., and D. H. Easer. *For Women Only: Chinese Herbal Formulas.* New Canaan, Conn.: Keats Publishing, 1994.

A discussion of Chinese herbal therapies for women's health problems, with fifty-three tried-and-true formulas for twenty-one female ailments, including uterine and breast cancer, menstrual problems and infertility, and other conditions usually treated with surgery and drugs.

Hsu, H. Y., and C. S. Hsu. *Commonly Used Chinese Herb Formulas with Illustrations.* Los Angeles: Oriental Healing Arts Institute, 1980.

A detailed presentation of traditional Chinese herbal formulas, listed by therapeutic categories, with information on history, effects, indications, and variations for each formula, with Chinese anatomical illustrations.

Hsu, H. Y., and W. Peacher. *Shang Han Lun: Well-Spring of Chinese Herbal Medicine.* New Canaan, Conn.: Keats Publishing, 1994.

A translation of and commentary on Chang Chung-ching's classical herbal canon, *Discussion of Fevers and Flus*, with contemporary interpretations.

Hunnan Health Committee. *A Barefoot Doctor's Manual* (Chinese Paramedical Handbook). Philadelphia: Running Press, 1997.

A field manual for paramedical practice in mainland China, combining traditional Chinese methods of diagnosis and therapy with modern Western technology and pharmaceutical therapy; a practitioner's guide to the New Medicine in Asia, blending the best of East and West.

Kaptchuk, T. J. *The Web That Has No Weaver.* Chicago: Congdon and Weed, 1983.

A thorough explanation of the basic concepts and classical terminology of traditional Chinese medicine, presented in both subjective and scientific terms of contemporary Western thought, with extensive appendices on traditional Chinese diagnosis; the author received his doctorate in Oriental Medicine at the Macao Institute of Chinese Medicine.

Keys, J. D. *Chinese Herbs.* Boston: Charles Tuttle, 1976.

Individual monographs on the major herbs used in Chinese herbal medicine, including information drawn from both classical Chinese sources and modern Western science, with illustrations and Chinese characters for each entry.

Lu, H. *Chinese System of Food Cures*. New York: Sterling Publishing, 1986.

A handbook of traditional Chinese nutritional therapy, with explanation of the Five Elements, Yin-yang, and other classical parameters in diet, plus specific nutritional remedies for various conditions.

Maciocia, G. *The Foundation of Chinese Medicine: A Comprehensive Text for Acupuncturists and Herbalists*. London: Churchill Livingstone, 1989.

A detailed general reference and practical guide to the clinical applications of acupuncture and herbs in traditional Chinese therapeutics, clearly elucidated for the Western reader.

————. *Tongue Diagnosis in Chinese Medicine*. Seattle, Wash.: Eastland Press, 1987.

Explanation of various facets of tongue analysis in traditional Chinese diagnosis, including color, texture, and zones, with guidelines for self-diagnosis.

Mann, F. *Acupuncture: The Ancient Chinese Art of Healing*. London: Heinemann, 1971.

A history and basic introduction to Chinese acupuncture as a treatment for disease, with simple explanations of terms and concepts.

————. *Acupuncture: Cure of Many Diseases*. London: Heinemann, 1971.

A sequel to Dr. Mann's first book, with further discussions of how acupuncture functions as a cure for various types of disease.

————. *The Meridians of Acupuncture*. London: Heinemann, 1974.

Detailed descriptions of each of the major organ-energy meridians used in acupuncture, including symptomatology, branch channels, related tissues of the body for each meridian, psychological aspects, and other facets, with a complete chapter on each meridian.

————. *The Treatment of Disease by Acupuncture*. London: Heinemann, 1974.

A point-by-point analysis of the functions and characteristics of all the major acupuncture points on the twelve primary organ-energy meridians, plus an alphabetical section on the treatment of specific diseases and symptoms by acupuncture.

Mowrey, D. *Herbal Tonic Therapies*. New Canaan, Conn.: Keats Publishing, 1993.

A highly informative scientific discussion of the tonic category of herbal medicine, focusing on potent preventive tonics for the nervous, circulatory, digestive, sexual, and immune systems, with well-documented data and detailed references of sources, written by one of America's leading authorities on herbal science.

———. *Next Generation Herbal Medicine*. New Canaan, Conn.: Keats Publishing, 1991.

A detailed scientific analysis of some important herbs used in herbal therapeutics, focusing on those now available in "guaranteed potency" form, including ginkgo, ginseng, *Echinacea*, and milk thistle, with extensive references from contemporary scientific resources.

———. *The Scientific Validation of Herbal Medicine*. New Canaan, Conn.: Keats Publishing, 1986.

A detailed scientific analysis of major herbs and formulas used in both traditional Chinese and Western herbal therapeutics, listed according to disease categories, with extensive footnotes on research references.

Nakamura, T. *Oriental Breathing Therapy*. Tokyo: Japan Publications, 1981.

A detailed explanation of the deep abdominal breathing techniques used in *chee-gung* self-health care practices, and their applications in curative and preventive therapy.

Needham, J. *Science and Civilization in China*. Vol. 2. New York: Cambridge University Press, 1962.

Historical milestones in the development of traditional Chinese medicine, with scientific interpretations of classical terms and concepts, from Needham's landmark encyclopedia of the history of Chinese sciences.

Needham, J. and G. D. Lu. *Celestial Lancets: A History and Rationale of Acupuncture and Moxa*. New York: Cambridge University Press, 1980.

A complete history and scientific explanation of acupuncture and moxibustion, with translations of classical references and modern scientific commentary.

Ni Hua-ching. *Strength from Movement: Mastering Chi.* Hong Kong: Seven Star Communications, 1994.

An authoritative exposition on *chee-gung* and its various styles of practice, the role of the body's "elixir field" energy centers, and the applications of *chee-gung* in health, longevity, and spiritual cultivation, written by one of the world's most venerable Taoist masters and a direct heir to a seventy-four-generation lineage of teachers.

Ni Maoshing. *The Yellow Emperor's Classic of Medicine.* Boston: Shambhala Publications, 1995.

A new translation of the ancient Chinese canon of medicine, with insightful commentary and conceptual clarifications by the translator.

Ramholz, J. *Shaolin and Taoist Herbal Training Formulas.* Chicago: Silk Road Books, 1992.

A compilation of tonic herbal formulas traditionally used by Chinese martial artists and meditators to cultivate and balance internal energy and enhance power, culled from classical references, with an index of Chinese characters for each formula.

Read, B. E. *Chinese Materia Medica: Animal Drugs.* Taipei: Southern Materials Center, 1976.

A translation of entries on Chinese medicinal products derived from animals, including domestic and wild monkeys and rodents, and human parts such as hair, bones, and urine, based on Li Shih-chen's classic pharmacopeia.

————. *Chinese Materia Medica: Avian Drugs (1932), A Compendium of Minerals and Stones (1936), Turtle and Shelifish Drugs (1937).* Taipei: Southern Materials Center, 1977.

A translation of entries on medicinal products derived from birds, shellfish, and minerals, based on Li Shih-chen's Ming dynasty compendium.

————. *Chinese Materia Medica: Dragon and Snake Drugs (1934), Fish Drugs (1939), Insect Drugs (1941).* Taipei: Southern Materials Center, 1977.

A translation of entries on medicinal products derived from reptiles, fish, and insects, based on Li Shih-chen's pharmacopeia.

Reid, D. *Chinese Herbal Medicine.* Boston: Shambhala Publications, 1987.

A concise introduction to the principles and practices of traditional Chinese medicine, focusing mainly on the herbal branch of therapy. Includes an illustrated guide to the nature and use of 200 Chinese herbs, drawn from original Chinese sources, plus some prescriptions for herbal formulas and recipes for herbal cooking.

————. *The Complete Book of Chinese Health and Healing (Guarding the Three Treasures).* Boston: Shambhala Publications 1994; and London: Simon & Schuster, 1994.

A sequel to *The Tao of Health, Sex, and Longevity,* focusing more on the aspect of energy in Chinese health care systems; includes introductory chapters on theoretical foundations, a section on major branches of therapy, information on energy pollution and energy medicine, descriptions of major Chinese patent formulas, herbal recipes, and list of mail-order suppliers.

————. *A Handbook of Chinese Healing Herbs.* Boston: Shambhala Publications, 1995.

An illustrated guide to the use, effects, and preparation of 108 Chinese healing herbs and thirty-six traditional formulas for home use, with a brief overview of basic terms and concepts, instructions for preparing herbs in the kitchen, a glossary of terms, an ailment index, and a list of suppliers.

————. *The Tao of Health, Sex, and Longevity.* New York: Simon & Schuster, 1989.

A comprehensive introduction to the major branches of traditional Taoist systems of human health care, including diet and nutrition, fasting, breathing, exercise, sexual yoga, meditation and internal alchemy, and longevity practices, combining traditional Chinese and modern scientific data.

Schwarz, J. *Human Energy Systems.* New York: E. P. Dutton, 1980.

A revealing analysis of the human energy system and its role in health and healing, including exercises for developing auric vision and an introduction to naturopathic energy healing methods.

Stuart, G. A. *Chinese Materia Medica: The Vegetable Kingdom.* Taipei: Southern Materials Center, 1976.

A translation of entries on Chinese medicinal products derived from plants, derived from Li Shih-chen's great Ming dynasty pharmacopeia, with an extensive commentary by the translator; an excellent reference guide for information on individual herbs in the Chinese pharmacopeia.

Teeguarden, R. *Chinese Tonic Herbs.* Tokyo: Japan Publications, 1984.

A detailed and informative guide to the most important tonic herbs used in Chinese herbal therapy, with scientific validation of traditional Chinese data on each herb discussed; includes a clear introduction to basic terms and concepts, guidelines for preparing herbal tonics at home, and appendices on sources, suppliers, and herbal categories.

Tin, Y. S. J. *The Book of Acupuncture Points.* Brookline, Mass.: Paradigm Publications, 1984.

An in-depth discussion of the therapeutic applications of the major acupuncture points, based on classical Chinese sources, with an introduction that gives an interesting account of the state of the art in China during the first half of the twentieth century.

Unschuld, P. *Approaches to Traditional Chinese Medical Literature.* Norwell, Mass.: Kluwer Academic Publishers, 1989.

An analytical interpretation of classical terms and concepts that appear frequently in traditional texts of Chinese medical literature, with selective translations.

Van Lysebeth, Andre. *Pranayama: The Yoga of Breathing.* London: Unwin, 1983.

This is one of the most complete and lucid explanations of *pranayama* in English, covering both the traditional aspects as well as modern scientific research that validates the ancient principles that govern the art and science of breath control. Some basic breathing exercises are also introduced.

Veith, I. *The Yellow Emperor's Classic of Internal Medicine.* Berkeley: University of California Press, 1966.

A translation of chapters 1–34 of this ancient canon of traditional Chinese medicine, including important commentaries by Wang Ping (762

CE) and Kao Pao-heng and Lin I (1078 CE), with an extensive introduction to basic terms and concepts by the translator.

Wiseman, N. *Glossary of Chinese Medicine.* Brookline, Mass.: Paradigm Publications, 1990.

A useful reference work of interpretive definitions of the major terms and concepts that appear most frequently in Chinese medical texts.

Waley, A. *The Way and its Power: A Study of the Tao Te Ching and its Place in Chinese Thought.* New York: Grove Press, 1958.

Arthur Waley's translation of this ancient Taoist text is considered by many readers to be the most beautiful of all English renditions. It is preceded by a lengthy introduction, which not only explains the importance of this classical work in Chinese thought but also paints a vivid picture of the entire edifice of traditional Chinese philosophy.

Wang, C. M., and L. T. Wu. *History of Chinese Medicine.* Taipei: Southern Materials Center, 1977.

A complete chronological history of traditional Chinese medicine from earliest antiquity to the first decades of the twentieth century, with biographical profiles of important physicians, discussion of the major texts, and commentary on the major medical milestones in Chinese history; illustrated and annotated.

Yang, J. M. *Chinese Qigong Massage.* Jamaica Plains, Mass.: Yang's Martial Arts Assoc., 1992.

A complete course in traditional Chinese massage, including basic concepts and theoretical foundations, as well as specific techniques and therapeutic applications; illustrated with schematic drawings and photographs; an excellent introduction to and practical manual for the massage branch of Chinese therapy.

————. *Muscle/Tendon Changing and Marrow/Brain Cleansing Chi Kung.* Jamaica Plains, Mass.: Yang's Martial Arts Assoc., 1989.

A translation of and detailed analytical commentary on Bodhidharma's two classic canons of *chee-gung, Yi Chin Ching* and *Hsi Sui Ching*; with historical background, philosophical foundations, and guidelines for personal practice.

————. *The Root of Chinese Chi Kung.* Jamaica Plains, Mass.: Yang's Martial Arts Assoc., 1989.

A comprehensive introduction to the field of Chinese *chee-gung,* including historical perspectives, scientific validations, therapeutic applications, and pointers for personal practice.

Zhang, Q. C. and Y. S. Hong. *AIDS and Chinese Medicine.* New Canaan, Conn.: Keats Publishing, 1994.

A detailed presentation of traditional Chinese medicine as a viable alternative treatment for AIDS, including herbs, acupuncture, *chee-gung,* and exercise, with clinical data from over 150 cases studies.

Index

Music, 42, 137
  therapeutic, 137

Native American views on health, 11
Nature, 1, 11
  as context for human life, 11
  as master template, 1
Navel (Gate of Life), 125–126, 131
Needles, types of acupuncture, 99–100, 108
Nervous system, 34–35, 127–128, 132
  chee-gung and, 127–128, 132
  immune response and, 128
  stress and, 127–128
Neuro-electric therapy (NET), 104–105
New Illustrated Manual on the Points . . . on the Bronze Man (Wang), 101
New Medicine, 20, 21
Nikolayev, Yuri (on hunger cure), 97
Nordenstrom, Bjorn (acupuncturist), 107
Nourishing energy (*ying-chee*), 33–34

Observation (diagnostic), 60
Organ meridians (*jing*), 35–36; 36
  See also Meridian system
Outlines and Divisions of Herbal Medicine (Li), 19
Overeating, 95–96

Pao Pu Tzu (Ko), 123
Paracelsus, 138
  vitalist philosophy of, 138
Pascal, Blaise, 134
Pasteur, Louis (germ theory), 48–49
Patent herbal formulas, 82–84
Patterson, Margaret (neuro-electric therapy), 104
Pediatric massage, 114–117
Pelvic floor, 130
  as second diaphragm, 130
Pericardium, 33
The Pharmacopeia of She Nung, 16
Piezoelectric effect, 137
Pranayama (breathing exercises), 123
Pranayama: The Yoga of Breathing (van Lysebeth), 37
Precious Recipes (Sun), 18, 86, 115, 122
Preventive health care, 3–5, 11
  food and, 3–4
  tonics and, 73

Psychoneuroimmunology (PNI), 9, 54, 132
  endocrine system and, 132
Psychoneuropathology, 54
Pulse diagnosis (*ba mai*), 61–62, 64

Questioning (diagnostic), 60

Rainbow Body (Tibetan yoga), 34
The Rainbow Diet (Cousens), 92, 93–94
Reflexology (foot massage), 113
  impotence and, 113
Reston, James, 107
Reverse abdominal breathing, 129

Salmanoff, A. (on respiratory function of diaphragm), 128–129
Schisandra, 74
Schumann resonance (earth's frequency), 127
  chee-gung and, 127
  healing and, 127
Schwartz, Jack (on chakra energy), 41
Sea of Energy (*chee-hai*), 125; 125
  navel and, 125–126
  See also Elixir Field (*dan-tien*)
Sea salt (*hai yen*), 72
Sedatives, 71–72
Self-acupressure points
  Ho gu (Valley of Harmony), 116, 119
  Nei guan (Inner Gate), 117
  Ren jung (Human Center), 117
  San yin jiao (Triple Yin Crossing), 116–117
  Tai chung (Supreme Thruster), 116, 118
  Yung chuan (Bubbling Spring), 117, 118
Self-massage, 117–119
  sexual (*dan hsiou*), 119
Seven Emotions (*chi ching*), 52–54
  modern manifestations of, 54
Shen (spirit, mind), 7–8
Shen Nung, Emperor (Divine Farmer), 13–14, 16, 77
Six Evils (*liu shieh*), 51–52; 51
  artificial forms of, 54–55
  Five Elemental Energies and, 51–52
Six Flavor Rehmannia Pills (*liu wei di huang wan*), 74, 82
Smith, Michael O. (on acupuncture/drug addiction), 105